Breath taking

Breath taking

Inside the NHS in a time of pandemic

RACHEL CLARKE

Little, Brown

LITTLE, BROWN

First published in Great Britain in 2021 by Little, Brown

1 3 5 7 9 10 8 6 4 2

A CIP catalogue record for this book
is available from the British Library.

Hardback ISBN 978-1-4087-1378-5
Trade paperback ISBN 978-1-4087-1377-8

Typeset in Bembo by M Rules
Printed and bound in Great Britain by
Clays Ltd, Elcograf S.p.A.

Papers used by Little, Brown are from well-managed forests
and other responsible sources.

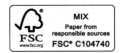

Little, Brown
An imprint of
Little, Brown Book Group
Carmelite House
50 Victoria Embankment
London EC4Y 0DZ

An Hachette UK Company
www.hachette.co.uk

www.littlebrown.co.uk

This book is dedicated to the memory of four members of staff at Oxford University Hospitals: Oscar King Junior, Elbert Rico, Philomina Cherian and Peter Gough.

Each lost their life to Covid-19 while doing their utmost to help others.

To date, over 600 NHS and care workers have suffered the same fate.

Heartfelt thanks to them all for their courage and selflessness.

Contents

Author's Note

The majority of these stories are told with the permission of patients, families and members of staff who kindly agreed to be interviewed for this book. I am extremely grateful to them all. Occasionally, an interviewee preferred me to tell their story using a pseudonym rather than their real name. In describing my own experiences, details of situations and the people I have met and cared for have been merged or altered in order to protect their confidentiality.

. . . perhaps the day will come when, for the instruction or misfortune of mankind, the plague will rouse its rats and send them to die in some well-contented city.

ALBERT CAMUS, *The Plague*

Prologue

He lies on hospital sheets, but he's drowning.

Behind closed doors, with neither fanfare nor drama, he's
been quietly drowning all night. The act of voicing distress –
alerting another human being to his plight – takes spare air
he no longer possesses. Wide mouth, wide eyes, face stunned
and stricken. The mask clamps down on skin slick with sweat.
His lips are grey, fingertips the colour of bruises. And though
the oxygen roars, the highest flow we can manage, it's still not
enough, not remotely.

My early-morning gasp, unlike his, can be heard. For weeks
now, every time I step out of the house, the signs of life astound
me. Spring in full tilt, all blossom and abandon. Skies so huge
and clean and blue they obliterate, if briefly, the hospital from
my mind. In this age of contagion, and only for moments, I
feel scrubbed clean of disease, disinfected. The man in the side
room stutters on.

Breathtaking

It's 7 a.m. While I'm on the motorway, the hospital will be stirring. Wan faces from night shifts will be emerging into light. With brains fogged and dim, blinking and yawning, colleagues will be dredging up sufficient energy to deliver the clean, crisp handovers those on the day shifts require. The new arrivals will be donning masks, scrubs and the necessary steeliness with which to endure the twelve hours to come. We are learning that minds as much as bodies require barricades these days.

There are drugs to be dispensed, temperatures to be taken, floors to be bleached, oxygen to be titrated, tea to be brewed, families to be updated, new decisions to be made in the cold light of morning about the patients now marooned between life and its extinction – like the man in the side room, alone and drowning.

I feel a little drunk in the car on sunshine and birdsong. Goodbye husband, goodbye children. Sleep on, my little locked-down loves. Don't drive Dad berserk, please. The deserted motorway feels faintly post-apocalyptic. Zombies, triffids, shambling corpses. All manner of B-movie foes could be stalking the hard shoulder, though in this war – as the newspapers like to frame it – we face an enemy too small to see. One thousand coronaviruses would barely span a human hair. Several trillion might just fill a pinhead.

As indices of apocalypse go, the number of free spaces in hospital car parks is a cast-iron measure of calamity. I pull up, disconcertingly close to the entrance to ED, the emergency department. My usual spot is some derelict tarmac tucked behind a row of uninhabited 1950s huts, condemned since the discovery of asbestos.

I open the boot of the car. No one in my family but me

is allowed in here. It's one thing to weigh your own risks of infection, but quite another to know that by going to work you might endanger those you love most dearly. One clean bag, one dirty. I sling each on to opposite shoulders, though if I'm honest, the distinction feels too slight to count as more than superstition. Still, you draw strength from where you can. One last glance towards the blue vault above. That warmth, those depths, the sheer spotlessness of empty sky. I breathe in deep, fill my lungs until my ribs splay wide. Anything feels possible beneath a sky like this. With every fibre straining back towards the sun and treetops, I lower my head and walk inside.

All the clamour and chaos of a hospital reception is long gone. No patients, no relatives, no jostling in the coffee queue, no shouting, no swearing, no flirting, no family spats, no crying babies, no bewildered octogenarians, no flummoxed visitors squinting and craning at the maps on the walls, just row upon row of empty seats in the normally overwhelmed atrium.

At the help desk, Molly looks bereft.

'Morning, doctor,' she smiles ruefully, a lover of hubbub now in charge of a ghost ship. One of our small army of hospital volunteers, she retired from her nurse's role well over a decade ago, but couldn't resist returning, a regular on the helpers' rota. No one knows quite how old she is now. 'The thing is,' she once told me, but only because I asked, 'I can't just stop helping people. That's why I became a nurse in the first place. It's who I am.'

I pause for a moment to say hello, keeping my requisite two metres' distance.

'Are you sure about still coming in, Molly?' I ask, raising an eyebrow. 'Without meaning to cast aspersions on your youthfulness, I'm guessing you're probably in the high-risk category if you catch it?'

She smiles. Her stack of photocopied guides to the layout of the hospital sits untouched on the desk beside her. I have observed her many times beaming confidence at new arrivals as they struggle to navigate the colour-coded signs to the endless wards and hubs and zones that sprout like bindweed in every direction. She has an uncanny ability to make everyone feel cared for – the secret elixir, I believe, of a hospital.

'How dare you!' she cries in mock indignation.

I grin but say nothing, and a second passes. Briefly, her breeziness wavers.

'I know the risks,' she says quietly, touching her name badge. 'We all do, don't we?'

I hesitate, glancing down at the text on the badge. 'Hello, my name is Molly. Can I help you?' it asks. Most definitely, is the answer. Indeed, without the hundreds of volunteers like her, the hospital would flounder. I know she loves her role, finds it meaningful, important. But the idea that her selflessness might end up being the death of her is surely a sacrifice too far?

'I guess I think of it like this,' I suggest, trying to put myself in her shoes. 'You're needed. The hospital needs you. But wouldn't it be better to take some time off now, rather than get infected and risk never returning?'

'Hmph,' she retorts, as if dismissing a small child. 'Aren't you late?'

She's right, I am. Handover is starting. I run to the toilets, strip off my jeans, pull on my scrubs and rush straight to the emergency assessment unit, the EAU.

The senior medical registrar is beginning his account of the night take. Patients have been delivered by ambulance to our doors thick and fast. The take — a tiny team of two or three doctors responsible for admitting new patients overnight — have assessed every one and made a crucial judgement: can they go home or are they sick enough to require admission? Whether they like it or not, doctors wield a God-like authority, for these are decisions with fatal implications.

Twenty or so of us have now assembled, too many to maintain strict social distance in a room this size. We shuffle and jostle in awkward estrangement, like identically poled magnets, each repelling the other. We know full well that hospitals are infection hotbeds. Any of us — the very people upon whom we most rely, our comrades in action — may unknowingly harbour the virus.

Sam, the med reg at the helm last night, has a reputation for toughness. Bespectacled, crooked-nosed and prematurely balding, he's part thug, part absent-minded professor. He cannot abide imprecision and rambling, but when his juniors need help — when a patient is in trouble — there is no one more calm or supportive. Without a hint of emotion, his terseness masking what must be bone-deep exhaustion, he rattles through the night's admissions. The same bleak story, over and over.

'Charles S. Sixty-one. Fever, breathlessness. Bilateral infiltrates on chest X-ray. Covid swab sent. Stable on 4 litres. Full escalation.

'Maureen W. Eighty-three. Fever, breathlessness, confusion. Bilateral infiltrates on chest X-ray. Covid swab sent. Desaturating on 15 litres. Ward-based care. Not for ITU [intensive therapy unit].

'Simon R. Forty-five. Fever, cough. Bilateral infiltrates on chest X-ray. Covid swab sent. ITU reviewing now. Already needing 6 litres.'

The names go on. The same symptoms, the same X-rays, the same need for extra oxygen. The same numbers that to medics signal lives in the balance. Of the score of patients admitted overnight, only a handful are believed not to have coronavirus. The youngest victim, aged thirty-five and pregnant, has already been transferred to intensive care.

But where, we keep thinking, is everyone else? The people with heart attacks, strokes, kidney stones, bleeding stomachs? Coronavirus hasn't merely overwhelmed the department, it has somehow displaced from the NHS the thousand and one additional reasons to be rushed on a trolley through the locked-down dark, sirens screaming, blue lights flashing, your stricken brain or heart or guts demanding our most urgent attention. Except it can't have done. We know this, it's not possible. And so, in the backs of our minds the missing dimly congregate, the people hiding out at home, lying low, keeping quiet, fearing hospitals have mutated from places of cure into modern-day plague sites, waiting and hoping for their pain to pass.

But a brain can hold only so much. Our focus is on Sam, who now reaches the end of his list, slowly pushing his glasses back above the bridge of his nose to signal he has nothing more to say. The normal banter of a handover – always inappropriate, frequently scatological and much loved by a tribe whose day job entails uncomfortable proximity to human suffering – is singular by its absence. No one feels very much like laughing just now. Doctors are dispatched in every direction, setting off with determined strides and sober expressions.

Briefly, my eyes meet Sam's. We've known each other since

medical school, stumbled through our first weeks together as petrified new doctors. In all that time, the trials and tribulations, I can't remember him looking this exhausted. Before leaving, I nod in his direction.

'Standards, Sam. You do realise you're wearing one grey sock, one blue?'

He frowns, glances down, then looks up in surprise. 'Oh dear. Am I letting the side down on compassionate excellence?'

We both crack a smile.

'Come on,' I admonish him. 'At least make an effort to be half full about it. Personally, I see your socks as disruptive innovation, Sam.'

He laughs. Our hatred of NHS management jargon was spawned in our first ever hospital induction when a man in a suit told us we were not being inducted but rather 'onboarded' since this was no run-of-the-mill induction at all, this was something bigger, better, full of dazzle and panache – an onboarding, whatever that meant, of the newest members of the corporate family. I remember stifling a laugh at Sam's levitating eyebrow.

As Sam wearily waves and hauls himself to bed, I set off towards the man in the side room. His name, I learned in handover, is Winston Potter. He is eighty-nine years old. Although we haven't met, I already know he is perilously ill. Despite the highest flow of oxygen we can deliver through a face mask, he is breathing at a rate of forty breaths per minute, two or three times the norm. I choose not to imagine what that must feel like.

A thick red stripe, freshly painted on the floor I'm crossing, dispatches me in Winston's direction. In just over a week, the hospital has been carved up into 'zones' of red and blue.

Although euphemisms hint at what constitutes 'red' – the signs in our newly merged ED and EAU coyly refer to the 'Respiratory ED', for example – everyone who works here knows this is code for coronavirus. An entirely new department, reconfigured in days, now exists to try to manage the onslaught of patients presumed or known to be infected. The visual metaphors could not be more explicit. Red is for danger, alert, blood and doom: this particular brick road leads to no Emerald City but a populace that fights for air, united in its hunger for oxygen.

Winston arrived twenty-four hours ago. Before I can enter the ward where he lies, I need to mask up. In theory, the masks we all wear – paper thin, though reinforced with a water-resistant coating – will prevent the virus from contaminating our mouth or nose, even when a patient coughs in our direction. I press the metal strip on the top of the mask hard on to my nose and cheekbones, endeavouring to mould it into a fit that is approximately airtight. It feels feeble, insubstantial, but it is all we have, and something is better than nothing.

In personal protective equipment (PPE), everything is hotter, stickier and more stifling than you'd like. Even breathing takes more effort. Voices are muffled, smiles obscured. Sweat starts trickling into your underwear. Behind our masks, we strain to hear each other speak and are forced to second-guess our colleagues' expressions. Being protected entails being dehumanised.

I track down Winston's nurse to find out her view of him. She looks run ragged, overwhelmed by what her ward has become. Not good, she tells me. He's frightened. Struggling. Sons are on their way in. This means his doctors have already concluded the worst, for only those judged to be imminently dying are permitted the mid-pandemic luxury of visitors.

Hastily, I trawl Winston's hospital record. I'm hunting for a glimpse of the man he used to be before coronavirus so violently reduced him. This morning's car radio lingers in my mind. Listening to the politicians and journalists talk – loftily, from afar, an Olympian perspective – coronavirus feels like a mathematical abstraction, an intellectual exercise played out in curves and peaks and troughs and endless iterations of modelling. But to us, the pandemic is a matter of flesh and blood. It unfolds one human being at a time. And when the statistics threaten to throw me off balance – this unprecedented number of deaths for peacetime – I try to keep things as small as I can. Winston used to work in the local glass factory. His wife died six months ago. Their sons are called Michael and Robert.

Over my mask, I layer on more protection. Apron, gloves and visor next, the minimum with which we approach our patients. Now my name badge is hidden from view and my eyes – the only part of my face still visible – are obscured by a layer of Perspex. So much for the healing presence of the bedside physician. Draped in this lot, I scarcely look human.

Entering the antechamber to Winston's side room, I'm dismayed to discover his sons are already here. Someone has helped them into their own protection, but one mask, I can see, is on inside out and both men look limp and bewildered.

'We don't know how close we're allowed to get to him,' says one.

'Can you tell us how long he has?' asks the other, in a voice made hard by fear.

I fight for a second to maintain my composure. All those arcs and sweeps and projections and opinions – the endless, esoteric, disorientating debates about whether flattening or crushing the curve is more desirable – arrive, in the end, at precisely this point, this moment of concrete simplicity. Six feet away, a father, a man I am yet to lay eyes on, is dying of a disease only named a month ago. His sons, trussed up in rubber and plastic, have turned to me, a total stranger with neither a face nor a name, for guidance. They don't even know I'm a doctor.

'Hello Michael, Robert,' I say warmly, though doubtful the warmth will carry. 'My name is Rachel. I'm one of the doctors caring for your father. Forgive me for not knowing which of you is which.'

'I'm Michael,' says the brother with the stony edge to his voice. 'No one's told us anything. Can he even hear us?'

Everything about this is wrong. The physical barriers between us – and between these sons and their father. The fact that they are feeling abandoned and scared. The hard and jarring words that conceal their rising panic. The glaring need – which can't be met – to rip off the masks and gloves and shake hands, sit down, read each other's expressions and begin, inch by inch, to cross the gulf that divides us.

'I'm sorry to hear that, Michael,' I begin. 'I'm going to try and answer all your questions in as much detail as I can, but would you mind if I assessed your father first? I'm just keen to make sure he doesn't need anything urgently.'

Two masks glance at each other, then nod reluctant assent. The sons step aside to allow me in closer and there, palms turned upwards, chest heaving and trembling, is Winston, spread-eagled in tangled cotton. An intravenous line drips antibiotics into one arm. A catheter drains urine the colour of mud into a bag left lying on the bedclothes. His legs, thin as bones, are twitching and scything. His fingers claw the air as though straining for a ledge to cling on to. The only part of his body not in motion, I realise, are his eyes which stare, white-rimmed, fixed vertically upwards.

The radio crosses my mind again. The language of war has been rife this pandemic but never more so than now, with the Prime Minister rushed recently to intensive care where he too is being treated for coronavirus. Since then, battle tropes have dominated the national conversation. Cabinet members assure us the PM will beat the disease because he's a fighter, as though survival is somehow a test of character, a matter primarily of valour. The reality, of course, is more banal. People do not die from this illness, or from any other, because they lack grit. Nor do they live through sheer pugnaciousness.

I look down at the bedsheets, stained with sweat, and the coil of limbs squirming in fear. It could not be plainer to anyone here that Winston is no participant in a battle. He is, instead, merely the battlefield. His body, worn out to begin with, is being quietly, methodically disposed of. And character has precisely nothing to do with it. It never does in the real world of the hospital where the good, the bad, the brave and the timid all kneel alike before cancers and microbes.

I move closer. Speaking loudly to be audible above the thrum of the oxygen, I say his name. Nothing. No flicker of response. Still closer. Again: 'Winston.' His eyes remain locked on the ceiling. I can feel those of his sons fixed on me.

In an era when even breathing the same air as your patient is heavy with risk, physical contact is permitted only when strictly necessary. I observe the muscles on Winston's neck, bulging to drag a little more air into his waterlogged lungs, and I am as certain as I am of anything in medicine that touch in this moment is essential.

Gently, I take his hand in both of mine. His pulse flutters so faintly, it is barely there. The blood in his fingertips has been purged of oxygen, transforming its colour from red to sludgy blue. No warmth from his flesh creeps through my gloves into mine. I am holding the hand of a man who is dying and who knows it as surely as I do. Here and now, a virus so primitive it scarcely qualifies as life is in the act of taking my patient's breath away.

I squeeze Winston's fingers, repeat his name once again, and now, at last, his eyelids flicker. Our gazes meet for the first time.

'Are you in any pain?' I ask.

A barely perceptible shake of his head. But when I ask if his breathing is distressing, he manages to nod.

'In just a moment, we'll help your breathing,' I promise. I go on, a vital question: 'Are you afraid?'

He nods a second time, and in turn I make a second promise. 'I'm going to ask the nurses now to bring you an injection which will help you relax and help your breathing.'

A final nod and then, just before turning to his sons, I lean closer still: 'Winston, Michael and Robert are here. They're going to sit with you now until the nurse comes.'

I straighten up from the bedside. I note the moisture glinting beneath the brothers' visors.

'Would you like to pull up these chairs?' I ask them. 'You can sit as close as you want, you can hold hands, you can say anything. Your dad needs some medicine to help his breathing, so I'm going to ask the nurses to give him something now – and then we can talk. Is that OK? I'll be back in a few minutes.'

Half an hour later, Winston has all the medications he

needs. With a little morphine and a small dose of sedative he has finally lost his look of undisguised horror. Winston's sons and I talk in low voices in the antechamber just outside his room. Although he appears to be sleeping peacefully, we need to assume he can hear every word and so I have taken his sons outside. Yes, I agree, time is short. Yes, he is probably in the last few hours of his life. I stress that I can no longer see any evidence of fear or suffering. That he is comfortable, peaceful, and that there is no reason now to assume he will not remain that way. It is Michael doing most of the talking, his voice now softer. But suddenly, almost desperately, his brother interjects.

'I don't want him to be a statistic!'

Robert knows full well — each of us in the room does — that tomorrow's televised press briefing will announce the precise number of people who have died from the virus today. Winston, almost certainly, will be among them. I see through Robert's eyes the colossal affront of someone you love — of all that your beloved has been and believed and meant to the world — being reduced to a numerical bit part in tomorrow's news headlines.

'He is *not* a statistic,' Robert says again, more resolutely.

Then he pauses.

In the bleakness and tenderness of the next four words, I think I understand for the first time the true cost of a pandemic.

'He's my best friend,' he murmurs.

When the once-in-a-century pandemic struck, it did not matter that it was predicted and expected, nor even that we had watched it before, playing out in multiplexes, paying money for the privilege of oohing and aahing over popcorn as big-screen contagions encircled the globe.

The idea of the end of everything – civilisation as we know it upending cataclysmically – is a much-loved staple of popular entertainment. Yet the real thing, an actual apocalyptic upheaval, seemed to catch the continents of Europe and America unaware. The pandemic's most shocking feature, you might argue, is how startled we all were as the realisation dawned: life as we knew it was temporarily over.

Asia, on the other hand, had seen lethal airborne plagues before. Here, coronaviruses had form. Recent outbreaks of SARS and MERS (the Severe Acute Respiratory Syndrome and Middle Eastern Respiratory Syndrome respectively) were each caused by a coronavirus hopping from animal to human hosts for the first time, with dramatic and deadly consequences. China, South Korea and Taiwan had been primed the hard way for another outbreak in a manner that, perhaps, for Britons in the sluggish depths of winter, seemed too outlandish to be taken seriously.

We ambled, half asleep, into disaster. In the first three months of 2020, perplexity drifted into mild concern that suddenly sheered into panic. Economies nose-dived. Schools and workplaces closed. Populations hid inside their homes. Whole societies shut down. In most people's living memory, no crisis had caused such global upheaval so swiftly and so comprehensively. The scale and pace of the pandemic were stunning.

By March, most of Britain had entered a state of suspended animation. With lockdown, time – the one commodity most of us crave more than anything – was suddenly available in enforced, unnerving abundance. A population in quarantine tried to manage its fears and listlessness using the unconventional strategies of baking bread and stockpiling toilet rolls.

Doctors, nurses and carers, on the other hand, were left reeling from frenetic activity. From top to bottom, with dizzying alacrity, the NHS transformed into a pared-down, single-minded, pandemic-focused field service. Psychiatrists, ophthalmologists, dermatologists and medical students were abruptly co-opted into pop-up intensive care units (ICUs). A conference hall mutated into a 4000-bed hospital. We were hastily taught how to wear our PPE, but half the items were missing, so we had to mime what we'd do with them. We tried not to think about catching coronavirus. The trickle of dead colleagues began.

As a palliative care doctor, I moved from the hospice to the hospital where the virus raged and surged like nothing we had seen before. In the early hours of the morning when I couldn't sleep, I'd creep downstairs so as not to wake my husband. Pacing the kitchen and tapping a keyboard became a kind of nocturnal therapy. Sometimes I would write until dawn. The gulf, I found, between the radiance of spring outside the hospital and the dying we witnessed within was both too great to convey to non-medical friends and family, and something I felt unable to inflict on them. The laptop, at least, enabled venting. Writing was an anchor. It helped distil my fears.

Later, when looking back over my insomniac's diary, I discovered that what I had thought was an unrelenting stream of death and darkness was in fact illuminated by pinpricks of light. People began to organise, street by street, village by village, to make sure that their most vulnerable neighbours, those self-isolating alone at home, were safe and fed and kept from harm. Teachers started using empty school science labs to fashion homemade protective visors for frontline staff. Rainbows sprang up on doors and in windows, painted by children to

encourage healthcare workers. A ninety-nine-year-old soldier walking laps of his garden inspired the public to donate
£30 million to the NHS. The curtailing of human contact, it
seemed, was reminding us precisely how precious it was, and
just how far a little of it could go.

But the most vivid and enduring bursts of relief came thanks
to, not in spite of, the hospital. Amid the tensions, fatigue and
rising death toll, moments that could stop you in your tracks
abounded. Michael and Robert, Winston's two anguished sons,
provided one such example. Shocked and distraught, having
just been told by me that their father was dying, you might
imagine they could not think beyond their grief. Indeed, when
Michael suddenly turned on me, I steeled myself for the anger
to come. Hostility, frustration, perhaps even a diatribe on how
far from ideal our care of his father had been.

'You have to promise me something,' he insisted.

I thought I knew what was coming, an urgent plea. Do not
leave him like this. Do not let him die alone. Instead came the
words which haunt me still.

'You have to promise me you'll make sure you don't catch
it. You, the nurses, all of you here. You have to make sure you
keep safe and don't catch it. I don't want any of you getting it
and going through what he is. Promise me.'

I stared at Michael. In this moment of torment, his father's
body breaking down but feet away, he had found it within himself to look beyond his own pain towards a wardful of doctors
and nurses he didn't even know.

I promised. How could I not? And I realised that what was
truly breathtaking about this pandemic was what it revealed
about the human beings to which it laid claim. 'Apocalypse' – a

term widely used to describe the early months of the pandemic – is typically a shorthand for the end of the world as we know it. But its etymology – the Greek word *apokalypsis* – means not a catastrophe but an unveiling, a revelation. Amid the devastation and upheaval of a genuine apocalypse, structures and certainties may be blown away, but hidden truths are revealed as well.

Above all – and contrary to my expectations – becoming a pandemic doctor was revelatory. The crisis has undeniably revealed sweeping truths about social and ethnic inequalities, class divisions, global interconnectedness and the fact that our society's most vital key workers were, and remain, among the lowest paid and least empowered. Historians will dissect these issues for years to come. My revelations were about people. I learned from ward to ward, from bedside to bedside, paying meticulous attention to one human being and then another. I discovered how to distinguish what we absolutely cannot do without from what is really, in the end, superfluous.

This book spans the four-month period from New Year's Day to the end of April 2020. Most of it is based on notes I wrote while in the eye of the storm, amid a national outpouring of uncertainty, grief and fear. The month of April was particularly gruelling. At the peak, a thousand deaths a day. I can still scarcely bring myself to write that, let alone comprehend it. There is something valuable, I believe, in attempting to document the rawness of this time. It was messy and ugly and overwhelming. Sometimes I could barely understand or name my emotions, let alone make claim to any wisdom.

There will be definitive accounts of the pandemic to come, but this is a snapshot, written fast and furiously. It depicts life, death, hope, fear, medicine at its most impotent and also at its finest, the courage of patients in enormous adversity, the stress of being torn between helping those patients and endangering your spouse and children, the long, fretful nights ruminating over whether the PPE you wear fits the science or the size of the government stockpile. I needed, I think, to take a stand with my pen and simply say: I was there. I have seen it, from the inside. I know what it was like. Here, with all its flaws and its inherent subjectivity, is my testimony. Make of it what you will.

I am exceptionally grateful to the hospice and the NHS trust where I work for supporting me in interviewing patients, relatives and other members of staff in order to piece together a deeper understanding of the experiences we have collectively endured. The book in no sense represents my employers' views, nor did they ever seek to influence my editorial independence. Thank you, Katharine House Hospice and Oxford University Hospitals NHS Foundation Trust, for believing this book could be positive. And thank you, all those individuals who entrusted me with their stories.

There is one thing I have learned above all this year. It is a conclusion I would like to sing from the rooftops. The NHS rose to the challenges magnificently. Not perfectly – certainly not – but with unstinting resolve to do its utmost for patients. Every single day, the grit and devotion of colleagues astounded me. In the eleven years I have practised as a doctor, I have never been prouder of nor more humbled by the NHS and its people. Faltering, fumbling, tenacious, undaunted, this is medicine in the time of coronavirus.

1

Pneumonia of Unknown Cause

*With infinite complacency men went to and fro over this
globe about their little affairs, serene in their assurance of their
empire over matter.*

H. G. WELLS, *The War of the Worlds*

The first day of the third decade of the twenty-first century
breaks softly over my speck of the globe. No ice on the wind-
screen, no frost on the road. Dawn emerging gently, in smudges
of grey. I stand on the doorstep in the cold, clean air and consider the robin considering me, head tilted, a few feet away.
Half an ounce of feathers and fight, its breast as bright as fire.

I grin. Hello, robin. Happy New Year.

The children are still sleeping, the babysitter's here and my
husband, a pilot, is destined for China. I have matters of life
and death to attend to, though today – unconventionally for a
doctor – these hinge primarily not on drugs and technology
but on the fortunes of Chelsea Football Club.

In Katharine House, the hospice where I work in rural

19

Oxfordshire, Christmas tinsel still glitters and donated tubs of chocolates and biscuits are piled high. People often flinch at the thought of palliative medicine, imagining a world full of dread and despair, all hope sucked away by death's proximity. Yet the hospice is strikingly beautiful. Its rooms are bathed in natural light from skylights and floor-to-ceiling French windows. In the fields outside, oak trees have endured for centuries, a perennial counterpoint to human impermanence. There are goldfinches, woodpeckers and great crested newts in the gardens; spa baths, massages and homemade smoothies for patients to enjoy inside. Pets are welcomed, romantic date nights encouraged, and the drinks cupboard stashed with every conceivable treat – because sometimes a sherry is as potent as morphine. Life, despite everything, goes on.

In so far as it featured in my years at medical school, death was treated less as a natural and inescapable fate – the one, indeed the *only* experience we are all guaranteed to share – and more as an embarrassing secret. We spent those five years fixated on cure. You went to medical school to learn how to stop people dying. First, we committed to memory the myriad illnesses afflicting human beings, and next, we were taught how to fix them. Death was alluded to coyly, if at all, as though its very existence might somehow taint doctors with an unsavoury whiff of defeat. Small wonder we approached the wards with unease.

'Tell me about Steve,' I say to the nurses.

Two days ago, I learn, a man in his fifties arrived at Katharine House from a local hospital. Oxford University Hospitals NHS Foundation Trust comprises four main sites: three imposing tertiary referral centres – the John Radcliffe Hospital, Churchill

Hospital and Nuffield Orthopaedic Centre in Oxford – and a smaller district general hospital, the Horton General Hospital in Banbury. I have known and worked in these hospitals for over a decade and am fiercely proud of all they achieve.

Steve Williams had been brought by ambulance from the John Radcliffe. Once trim and fit, Steve had run his own business until mysteriously, a few months ago, he had found himself occasionally coughing while drinking. The minor irritation of a splutter upon swigging his morning tea soon progressed into something less easy to ignore.

'Your voice isn't right,' Tessa, his wife, told him gently one day. 'I'm finding it hard to understand what you're saying.'

Cajoled against his will towards his GP, Steve soon found himself prodded, poked, scanned and scrutinised by the most intellectual of all the hospital specialists – the neurologists – until one day he found himself pinned in shock to his chair as a diagnosis was dropped like a stone into still water.

Like 'cancer', the words 'motor neurone disease' have the power to stupefy. Life's meaning and arc – its onward trajectory – are swept away at a stroke. The sensation of life being stopped in its tracks is one from which some patients never recover.

In Steve's case, the intricate muscles controlling his speech and swallow were inexorably weakening. By early summer, he had a device in place enabling him to be fed by a tube directly into his stomach. By late autumn, he relied on Tessa to suction excess fluid from his mouth and throat to prevent him from choking on his own saliva. By Christmas, his breathing was laboured and he could barely lift a pen. His mind still whirred, his imagination soared, but both were now essentially incarcerated.

Over Christmas, Steve had been rushed by ambulance to hospital, perilously close to respiratory failure. On Boxing Day, his breathing stopped altogether. A few seconds later, his heart ceased beating. Somehow, against the odds, the crash team's best efforts resurrected him from his cardiopulmonary arrest. Throughout his entire, rollercoaster admission, Steve was hell bent on one thing. On wasted legs, wobbling and weaving, he fought with every last breath to leave the hospital, a frail and doomed absconder. No one understood what propelled him.

When the paramedics drop Steve off at the hospice, he is, like many patients, disorientated and bewildered. Before entering his room, I prepare for a potential altercation. But to my surprise, sitting in an armchair beside a set of French windows is someone whose eyes coolly track my every move. I have the distinct impression it is me, not my patient, under scrutiny.

The muscles in Steve's neck are as warped and contorted as tree roots. His head teeters to one side like a trunk on the brink of being felled. Both shoulders are permanently hunched towards his ears, one hand has turned into a claw. The sheer effort of attempting to speak triggers spasms of jerking and yanking. It is as though Steve's muscles of speech can only be compelled into action by enlisting those of his entire upper torso – his deltoids, platysmas and sternocleidomastoids all quivering and twitching with exertion. As he nods and writhes, honking unintelligibly, I suspect the irony is lost on neither of us that the more he struggles to speak, the more obscured and impenetrable his words are.

Sitting next to her husband is Tessa, who takes over as a brisk, no-nonsense interpreter. She paints a bleak but familiar picture of overworked hospital doctors and nurses at Christmas. Across the country, when the seasonal pressures of winter flu collide with endemic NHS understaffing, it is painfully challenging to provide exemplary patient care. Through no fault of their own, staff can end up overwhelmed and exhausted. In the hospice, we are lucky enough not to face the same pressures. We have the luxury of time. I decide to risk a bold question.

'May I ask you something, Steve?' I say, looking directly at him. 'Do you ever feel frustrated that because you can't speak clearly, people don't always realise you have something important to say?'

'Yes!' he exclaims – it's half word, half yowl – but the passion and meaning are self-evident. It turns out that while in hospital Steve had had one simple desire: to do as he had done every Saturday since boyhood, when he would sit religiously next to his dad and watch Chelsea on the telly. Chelsea's Boxing Day match had been no ordinary fixture. It might, he'd known well, have been the final time he would ever watch his team play. Framed like that, those ninety minutes had meant everything.

Unable to communicate any of this, Steve had resorted to attempting to flee the hospital. Rage drove his withered legs into action. And though this break for freedom was an act of desperation, in the context of gagging day and night on your own saliva – of the end of your life so plainly approaching – it could hardly be seen as unreasonable.

Now, in the calm of his own room, all of that anger has gone. Through their attentiveness, the nurses who cared for Steve overnight have managed to make him feel heard. 'I have another extremely important question to ask you,' I announce solemnly. Steve raises a quizzical eyebrow. My pause is deliberately dramatic. Then: 'When are Chelsea next playing?'

A volley of booms fills the room – Steve's explosive version of laughter.

Their next match, it turns out, is today – New Year's Day – so we have no time to waste. It takes a surprising amount of negotiation to arrange emergency access to Premier League streaming, I discover, especially for a middle-aged mum whose idea of televised sport is watching Prime Minister's Questions. But here we are, at noon on the first day of the decade, with kick-off fast approaching. I didn't dare tell Steve in advance he could watch the match, for fear of being foiled by technology at the eleventh hour. So, it falls to his son to break the good news.

'Dad,' he grins. 'We've got a surprise for you. I'm here to watch the match with you.'

For a moment, Steve looks nonplussed. Then the room lights up with a grin of lopsided delight and thunderclap barks of mirth.

While I am prescribing emergency football matches, some 5500 miles away in central China another doctor is greeting the new year with an increasing sense of foreboding.

Li Wenliang is a thirty-three-year-old ophthalmologist practising in Wuhan Central Hospital. As you might imagine, doctors who choose to specialise in treating diseases of the eye tend to be meticulous observers. Anyone who takes miniature scalpels to the human eyeball – usually while their patients are awake and conscious – possesses an uncanny ability to gaze without flinching.

In a country where dissent can have grave repercussions, Li is sufficiently perturbed by unfolding events in his hospital to take to social media to warn his colleagues. His post to a group of old classmates from medical school alerts them to a mystery new disease in Wuhan Central. Seven people, he writes, are already in quarantine in his hospital with symptoms that look very similar to SARS. He urges his fellow doctors to wear protective equipment to prevent further infection.

In the early 2000s, SARS passed many Europeans and Americans by. The disease emerged in China in 2002 when a virus was transmitted from horseshoe bats to a cat-like mammal called a civet, and from civets in turn to humans. The pathogen, it emerged, was a type of coronavirus – a family of viruses known then to most doctors only as a cause of the common cold. But this one, a novel coronavirus, had never infected humans before and its effects were deadly. Without a vaccine, any form of treatment or previous exposure to the virus, nearly 10 per cent of those infected went on to die. Over half of those aged sixty-five and over did not survive their infection. Fortunately, the outbreak was stopped in its tracks after causing just over 8000 cases of infection and 800 deaths.

Like Li, several other doctors in Wuhan, an industrial city of 11 million people, are sufficiently afraid that SARS has resurfaced to risk incurring the wrath of the state themselves. 'Wash your hands! Face masks! Gloves!' another medic writes. To the fury of the local authorities, the smattering of posts from the medical profession are widely shared online, forcing the hand of Wuhan's health commission. At 1.38 p.m. on 31 December, it announces the detection of a cluster of 27 cases of a 'pneumonia of unknown cause' in the areas surrounding the city's seafood market. 'The disease is preventable and controllable,' the authorities add, with 'no obvious evidence of human-to-human transmission'. Their confidence is evidently not shared by Wuhan's clinicians.

The next day, while I am busy with my New Year's ward round, masked police officers and workers enclosed head-to-toe within fluid-repellent hazmat suits descend en masse on Wuhan's Huanan Seafood Wholesale Market. The market spans some twenty streets in the city. Long before dawn, the stallholders here have been piling high their fresh produce. Slabs of freshly slaughtered beef and pork hang from hooks above the butchers' counters. Scores of ducks with broken necks dangle upside down from their feet like colonies of mangled bats. The air is dense with the scents of fish, fruit, vegetables, spices and the tang of blood.

Huanan is a wet market – so-called after the melting ice that keeps its seafood fresh and the stallholders' technique of sloshing produce with cool water, while hosing slop and detritus into gutters. Its clatters and yells and general rowdiness include squawking, squeaking, barking and yelping, for the freshest produce of all is still warm and wriggling until, on handing over your coins, its throat is cut there and then for you.

There is a notorious corner of Huanan market, a wild animal section where over a hundred species, both live and slaughtered, can be purchased. Live wolf pups, scorpions, foxes, koalas, hedgehogs, golden cicadas, salamanders, peacocks, beavers, snakes and lizards are just some of the creatures available. In addition, various prized parts of some animals – such as crocodile tails, bellies, tongues and intestines – are all on sale separately.

Conditions here are cramped and filthy, the stench overpowering. To save space, the wildlife is stacked up high in cages, squirrels on badgers, turtles on bats, bamboo rats on civets. Amid the snarling and snapping of impounded animals, a gravitational trickle of bodily fluids – saliva, faecal matter, blood and urine – takes place in slow drips and sudden spatters, from cage to cage, species to species, animal to human.

When the police arrive on New Year's Day, they weave a perimeter of tape around the kiosks and stalls, ordering the owners to leave. The men in hazmat suits move in, depositing samples from tables and gutters in sealed specimen bags, systematically hosing down every street and disinfecting every surface.

As word reaches Li Wenliang that the market has been shut down, perhaps he allows himself a glimmer of optimism. His four-year-old son knows nothing of viruses and his wife is pregnant with their second child. The future brims with hope. But any relief is short-lived. Four days after he tries to warn his colleagues, the security forces turn up unannounced at Li's house one night, detaining him for 'spreading false rumours'. He is forced to sign a humiliating police document admitting he has breached the law and 'seriously disrupted social order'. A few days after the authorities release him, Li is back at his hospital, operating on a woman's eyes to correct her glaucoma. Later, it will transpire that she works at the seafood market. Unbeknown to both doctor and patient, she is brewing a viral infection.

In January 2020, novel coronaviruses are nowhere on my mind. Like everyone working in the NHS, I am steeled for a home-grown catastrophe. For no matter how many patients lie on trolleys in corridors, how many ambulances sit trapped on hospital forecourts, how many photos go viral of toddlers slumped on their parents' coats, receiving oxygen on the floor of a beleaguered A&E, nothing ever truly changes. These days, the annual NHS 'winter crisis' is both dreaded and reliable as clockwork.

The numbers are so large, and repeated so frequently, they have long been leached of their force: 17,000 hospital beds lost since 2010; only 2.5 beds per 1000 people in the UK, compared to three times that number in Germany; an NHS workforce so depleted it has unfilled vacancies for over 10,000 doctors and 40,000 nurses; and in social care – the NHS's much-neglected and impoverished sister – an eye-watering 120,000 unfilled vacancies.

Yet underlying these statistics are, of course, individuals. Patients – people – at their most exposed and vulnerable. NHS staff dread winter because nothing quite curdles the soul like pouring your all into a system at breaking point. Up close, the failures of care are the furthest thing from an abstraction. They assail you in the cries and whimpers of elderly patients with dementia abandoned on trolleys, in the sourness and sweat of the crumpled sheets in which a patient has just died, alone and unnoticed. They come in the form of verbal abuse from relatives at breaking point who turn on the doctors and nurses because we are there, the human face of all the underfunded dysfunction. They can make you want to cry or quit. You brush yourself down and carry on.

'How do you think it's going to be this time round?' a colleague asks me.

'Well, we don't seem to have been on black alert as much as usual,' I answer cautiously. 'Maybe flu hasn't hit as badly as people feared?'

For safety reasons – in order to manage surges in demand – hospital bed occupancy should sit below 85 per cent. Yet year round in today's NHS, occupancy is nearer 100 per cent. There is absolutely no spare capacity. The severity of a particular year's strain of seasonal influenza may thus spell the difference between keeping heads above water or full service implosion. A virus so tiny it requires an electron microscope to be seen can, in short, bring the NHS behemoth to its knees.

In fits and starts, news is trickling out of Wuhan and none of it is good. On 9 January, the world's first known fatality from the new virus occurs. A sixty-one-year-old man who regularly shopped at the seafood market dies in hospital after developing breathing difficulties and a raging fever. The same day, the first reports of the outbreak appear in the UK press.

'Are doctors and nurses treating patients, or family members, who have not had the same exposure to the source, also getting sick?' the head of the Wellcome Trust, Sir Jeremy Farrar, asks in a measured piece in the *Guardian* newspaper. 'If the infection is not passing person to person, then the level of concern is somewhat reduced – although it can always happen later, and infections can change.'

Farrar has identified the crux of the matter: a virus's lethal potential is intimately linked to how easily it passes from one host to another. Thus far, the Chinese authorities have insisted there is no clear evidence of human-to-human transmission in Wuhan, but cases in the city are rising exponentially and many have no link to the seafood market or to its live animal produce.

Several days after Farrar's remarks, Li Wenliang is rushed to his hospital's intensive care unit. The viral culprit in Wuhan has just been identified. Like the SARS outbreak in which one in ten of those infected died, this too, it turns out, is caused by a novel coronavirus. The high fever and compulsive cough that Li recently developed at home are now accompanied by a life-threatening shortness of breath. His lungs are beginning to fail.

It takes until 20 January for China to concede what doctors like Li observed from the outset, that human-to-human transmission is occurring. The authorities cite one example in which a single patient went on to infect fourteen healthcare professionals. With cases already being reported as far afield as Thailand, Japan, South Korea and the US, the admission is far from surprising to scientists. Borne on ships and planes, passing undetected from passenger to passenger, a microscopic assailant is circumnavigating the globe.

Two days later, in the UK, a committee of experts known as the Scientific Advisory Group for Emergencies (SAGE) meets for the first time to advise the government on the implications of the novel coronavirus. Cases have now leapt to 571 in China, with the official death toll standing at 17. The World Health Organization (WHO) stops just short of declaring the situation an international public health emergency, with its director-general, Tedros Adhanom Ghebreyesus, warning: 'Make no mistake. This is an emergency in China. But it has not yet become a global health emergency. It may yet become one.'

From now on, although the risk to the UK population is judged to be 'low', every flight from Wuhan will be monitored by public health officials. Passengers will be assessed for symptoms of coronavirus and quarantined if any are present. There are three flights a week from Wuhan to Heathrow. In the preceding fortnight alone, 2000 passengers from Wuhan have already entered the UK.

Nevertheless, the tone of an official communiqué sent out

from the Department of Health and Social Care to all NHS bodies is understandably soothing. 'The UK is well prepared for new diseases and our approach is kept under constant review,' it states, seeking to minimise panic. 'UK public health measures are world-leading and the NHS is well prepared to manage and treat new diseases.'

Predictably, the statement ignites lurid newspaper headlines. 'UK on Killer Virus Alert' screams one front page; 'Is the Killer Virus Here?' shrieks another. When I read them, I immediately recall a night several years earlier when I too found myself inwardly screeching in seventy-two-point capitals, while wrestling to maintain my external composure.

Back then, in 2014, a different virus was splashed all over the front pages. Ebola, a type of viral haemorrhagic fever, was running rampant across west Africa. The disease is highly infectious and has devastating potency, causing half of those infected to die. In its terminal stages, when patients are at their most contagious, they are prone to both internal and external bleeding. Victims may haemorrhage from their nose, ears, mouth and eye sockets. To me, the chances of an illness so remote – both geographically and in terms of my own experience – ever reaching Britain seemed fancifully slim. For all our global interconnectedness, what was happening in Guinea, Liberia and Sierra Leone felt as far flung as the moon. My imagination refused to stretch that far.

When several cases of Ebola emerged in the US and Spain, those of us in the hospital who might conceivably encounter a case ourselves were taught how to minimise our risks of infection with personal protective equipment – plastic boots, double gloves, gown, mask and visor. Even then, the precautions seemed excessive, our training dutifully undertaken without truly believing our lives might depend on it. It was only in the early hours of one Saturday morning that I learned, as the most junior doctor on-call for infectious diseases, how abruptly complacency can lurch into fear.

The call came from A&E. That evening a young man had walked into the department drenched in sweat and close to collapsing. He'd landed at Heathrow that day from a country adjacent to the main Ebola outbreak where, for a month, he had been visiting his extended family. Ordinarily with a traveller returning from that location, your first thought would be malaria. Statistically, it *should* be malaria. But with a smattering of Ebola cases in the region, the infection could not be ruled out.

'We really don't think it's likely. He was pretty hit and miss with his anti-malarials,' the A&E doctor told me. 'But when he arrives on your ward you might want to bear it in mind.'

With those words, I discovered how very like a virus fear can be. How viscerally it is felt, in the spine and the stomach, and how easily transmitted to others. In moments, fear had infected the length of the ward. The faces of the nurses tightened, the mood grew grim. Something dreadful and alien from far away – a sickness that surely only happened to other people, distant people – had as good as infiltrated the room.

This was what it felt like, I realised, to know that a fatal disease from another continent might be sweeping towards you, capable of striking any of you down. This was the pre-vaccination, precarious world of my grandparents' generation in which infectious diseases like smallpox, polio, diphtheria and scarlet fever terrorised Britain.

When the infectious diseases consultant called the ward to check in, the squirming in the pit of my stomach embarrassed me. 'Look, the likelihood of this being Ebola is so slight it's basically theoretical,' he reassured me. 'I'll come in right away if you'd like me to though? It's not a problem at all.'

I rebuked myself. Bloody drama queen. Just put the kit on carefully and check him like you would any other patient. Stop being pathetic.

'Not at all,' I answered in a voice that conveyed, I hoped, I had no need of hand holding. 'I'll let you know as soon as the malaria films are back.'

In the gloom of the ward at 3 a.m. we steeled ourselves for our patient's arrival. The nurse who would accompany the patient and me into his specially designated side room slowly exhaled. 'It's a bit like being in a movie, isn't it?' she commented. She was right. Standing there in our chin-to-floor gowns and gleaming white anti-Ebola wellington boots, we might have felt absurd had it not been for the fear needling the nape of our necks. Ebola had already jumped the species barrier from bats to humans. Was it really so implausible that its next leap might be on to us?

As we stood side by side, affecting nonchalance, I thought back to learning in medical school about the HIV epidemic. How horrified I'd been to discover that then, in the 1980s, many hospitals in New York simply turned away patients who were dying from AIDS, refusing to allow them to enter the building. Or that, even when a hospital did agree to admit them, patients would often have their food trays dumped on the floor outside their rooms or be left lying for hours in their own excrement by ward staff too scared to enter. How could those trained to heal, I'd naively thought, have behaved so inexcusably callously?

The power of contagion, I knew now, was the answer. My skin crawled in the semi-darkness. Images of bloodstained shrouds and bleeding eyeballs made me long to be anywhere but here. It felt shameful, a dirty secret, but my instinct to help was counterbalanced by another, equally potent – to flee.

By the time the young man arrived, a litre or two of intravenous fluid had done wonders. Alert, chatty and apologising profusely for the trouble he had caused, he certainly didn't look to be on the brink of exsanguination. My hands shook a little as I examined him, but my heart was already decelerating. Shortly afterwards, the lab rang through with the results of his blood tests. As suspected all along, he had malaria.

'There you go,' said my consultant when I called him. 'Of course it was never going to be Ebola. You can treat him as a straightforward malaria.'

On the ward, the fear receded, our smiles returned and we laughed away the collective dread that only hours earlier had felt so pervasive. Later, once safely back at home, I marvelled at our capacity for telling ourselves the stories we wish to hear. Those of us sufficiently lucky to inhabit rich nations can almost persuade ourselves we have banished biology. Our filtered, cocooned, air-conditioned existences are walled off from the contingencies of the natural world. We can control temperature, moisture, we can even make snow. As for plagues, droughts, floods and tempests, we can defy them all – or so we like to believe – with our brilliant minds and our dazzling technology. Survival of the fittest no longer applies when you can manipulate the world as adroitly as we do.

And then, at a stroke, the most minute of all forms of life manages to rupture this bubble of big talk and false comfort. Ebola – or so we fear – catches a plane, flies 4000 miles north, brings an A&E to a standstill and makes an inexperienced doctor's blood run cold. Suddenly, the natural world feels every bit as perilous and indomitable as it did a century ago, when microbes could lay waste to us all.

On 30 January, only days after its initial cautious optimism, the WHO revises its opinion of the novel coronavirus. With the death toll in China now standing at 213 – nearly ten times what it was a week earlier – the disease is officially declared a WHO Public Health Emergency of International Concern, one level of severity below a pandemic. France, Germany and Italy have all now announced their first cases.

Britain too is gripped by seismic upheavals. On 31 January, the *i* newspaper's front-page splash – 'UK's Leap into the Unknown' – could easily refer to the first two coronavirus cases just diagnosed on UK soil. Instead, it describes a political milestone, our departure from the European Union. Yet Brexit is about to be wiped from our minds, compared to the calamity to come.

2

The Might of Tiny Things

A virus is a piece of bad news wrapped in protein.

SIR PETER MEDAWAR, *Aristotle to Zoos:*
A Philosophical Dictionary of Biology

Two photos of one doctor, each taken days apart, tell an indelible story of power and impotence. In the first, the man's composure is striking. His hair is neatly trimmed, his skin smooth and youthful as he stares directly into the camera. Wire-rimmed spectacles sit atop two surgical masks – this is someone taking absolutely no chances. Adjacent to his ear, an anatomical cross-section of a human eye peeks out in poster-sized dimensions from the wall behind him. A sliver of conjunctiva, cornea and iris – then the lens, half obscured by the polypropylene bulge of the well-intended yet ill-fitting outer mask.

The second photo is the one I can't tear my eyes from. Now the doctor lies prostrate on white hospital sheets, face coated in sweat, dark hair sodden, cheeks flushed with fever. In a word, we would say he looks 'toxic' – the unmistakable stigmata of an infection so severe it makes the entire body appear poisonous. Beneath the plastic mask delivering high-flow oxygen, unruly tufts of stubble sprout from his jaw and upper lip. He has clearly been here for some time.

In the early hours of 8 February, Li Wenliang's image glows from my phone with an almost hallucinatory intensity. Wuhan Central Hospital's ceiling lights are reflected from his pupils into mine. We are both thousands of miles and inches apart. Despite freedom of expression being fiercely suppressed in China, Li has chosen to upload these selfies on to the Chinese social media site Weibo – the doctor who refused to stay mute. I suppose when you have tried to sound a warning about a lethal new infection, then been summoned for a dead-of-night police reprimand, then been felled at a stroke by the same virus you forewarned about, the power of the authorities becomes less consequential. When your life hangs in the balance, what more can they actually take from you?

Li's eyes, I believe, are beaming reproach into mine. I see neither fear nor distress, despite his toxic sheen. He looks like a man who knows precisely the measure of his actions and their chain of potential reactions. Those eyes, I am certain, are urging us to act.

Even as his vitality ebbs away, Li's determination to speak out only grows. 'After I recover, I still want to return to the front line,' he tells one Chinese newspaper, the *Southern Metropolis Daily*. 'The epidemic is still spreading and I don't want to be a deserter.' He even speaks online from his hospital bed to the heretical (for China) *New York Times*. 'My older child is four years and ten months old,' he states. 'The younger one is still unborn, due in June. I miss my family. I talk to them by video . . . I started coughing on Jan. 10. It will take me another fifteen days or so to recover. I will join medical workers in fighting the epidemic. That's where my responsibilities lie.'

The recovery never comes. Li's image is lighting up the internet tonight because at 2.58 a.m. on 7 February – six days after the second photo was taken – he dies, one of 636 victims in China, so far, of the still unnamed coronavirus. In death, Li attains instant and worldwide martyr status, a symbol of fragile and unassuming resistance against the punitive might of a total-itarian state. An explosion of anger and defiance erupts online. The hashtag 'We want freedom of speech' begins trending on Weibo. Strident demands for democracy soar. Every time the authorities clamp down and erase all the posts linked to a particular hashtag, Weibo users simply create an alternative.

As my husband sleeps soundly beside me, my eyes begin to swim. I bite my lip as I stare at the clear-sighted ophthalmolo-gist who chose, for the sake of future patients, to reach out – to go viral – even as a virus laid claim to his life. He was young and healthy, a man in his prime. If doctors like Li are dying, I think, what exactly has arrived here in Britain? How many more deaths of healthcare workers are there to come?

From this moment on, I start to pay closer – almost ghoul-ish – attention to the details now emerging from Wuhan. The city was plunged into panic when, on 24 January, the day before Chinese New Year, a total lockdown was imposed on its 11 million citizens, sealing them inside the city with its as yet nameless plague. Since then, stories and video footage have emerged online of overwhelmed hospitals turning patients away, relatives screaming for help for their loved ones, medics on street corners openly weeping. Government posters spring up all over the city, telling people: 'Don't go outside or gather in crowds. Wash your hands. Don't believe rumours or spread them. Have faith, this hardship is temporary.'

But is it? Photos of bodies lying motionless on the pavements outside Wuhan's hospitals are circulating on social media. Mounds of mobile phones are filmed outside crematoriums, where they have been piled high by undertakers too busy with corpses to know exactly what to do with handheld technology. As Fang Fang, an outspoken Chinese writer living in Wuhan, puts it: 'You begin to see things you never imagined humans were capable of.'

In Britain, the lurid upheavals of an unfamiliar Chinese city largely pass the population by. We are urged, somewhat tepidly, to wash our hands but otherwise life goes on undeterred. My husband, Dave, thinks I'm a raving hypochondriac to fret about weird diseases in distant parts of the world. 'Thank goodness your favourite meal isn't pangolin,' he replies as I try to engage him in the mortality rates of SARS and MERS.

'But you've been back and forth to China this winter,' I point out. 'Aren't you even slightly concerned?'

'It's my job,' he responds, the calm counterpoint to my excessive zeal. 'Travel is what pilots do. And no, I refuse to lie awake at night over something that will probably never happen.'

Dave deals with problems as they emerge, as opposed to squandering his energy on fruitless speculation. His attitude is more constructive than my obsessive midnight scrolling. But like Li Wenliang, whose online doctor groups hummed with anxious chatter long before the rest of China caught up, my medic friends and I are now nervously messaging each other about what is – or may be – to come. Our trepidation only increases when, on 10 February, the health secretary

Matt Hancock announces that the novel coronavirus 'now constitutes a serious and imminent threat to public health'. In keeping with the gravity of this threat, the state will give doctors 'strengthened powers' to detain and forcibly quarantine people suspected of having the virus.

Quarantine. I have always dimly associated the word, I realise, with gleaming images of starkness and whiteness. Patients hygienically sealed within state-of-the-art plastic bubbles by scientists in absurdly pristine lab coats. It's all Hollywood nonsense, of course. Actual quarantine, as my nocturnal reading habits make abundantly clear, is the fug of fear and sweat and ever-present contagion. It's the rice running out, the supermarket shelves laid bare, the stench of rotten fish from the abandoned seafood market, the pleading and sobbing outside a hospital's closed doors.

I try to imagine being sequestered inside my house, my village, my county and beyond, with real or metaphorical black crosses freshly daubed on our front doors. It would be the ultimate postcode lottery, this enforced and brutal intimacy of the healthy and the damned, living from minute to minute, hour to hour, cheek by suppurating jowl. I grew up simultaneously repelled and enthralled by teachers' tales of the Black Death ravaging medieval Britain. Yet still I find the notion of quarantine here today inconceivable – like revolutions, military coups, black widow spiders and tsunamis. The mortal computations of sacrificing some in order to save others who happen to live outside the *cordon sanitaire* feel too misplaced – too otherworldly – to grasp. Quarantine cannot apply to the citizens of Basingstoke and Bognor Regis. The idea of it is absurd.

On 11 February, the same day Matt Hancock expands upon

his quarantine plans to a packed House of Commons, the novel coronavirus is bestowed with a name. Naming, as anyone who has ever experienced the taunts of school bullies knows, can be an act of dominion or ascendancy, a way of flexing your muscles over that which you seek to control. Conversely, in *Call Them by Their True Names*, her collection of essays about naming as a means of seeing or revealing – of exposing things as they truly are – the American author Rebecca Solnit writes:

> When the subject is grim, I think of the act of naming as diagnosis. Though not all diagnosed diseases are curable, once you know what you're facing, you're far better equipped to know what you can do about it. Research, support, and effective treatment, as well as possibly redefining the disease and what it means, can proceed from this first step. Once you name a disorder, you may be able to connect to the community afflicted with it, or build one. And sometimes what's diagnosed can be cured.

Solnit is referring here to pernicious diseases of the socio-political kind – racism, misogyny, homophobia and the like – but her words might equally apply to medical taxonomy. The moment you label an illness, you change how it will be perceived. To name is to pay attention, to transform strangeness into familiarity, to hone your focus. In medicine, a name is the first step towards controlling the menace of a new threat to life, even if all that is really achieved is a linguistic illusion of control.

The WHO assigns the newest member of the coronavirus family the name SARS-CoV-2, which stands for 'severe acute respiratory syndrome coronavirus 2.' The infectious disease to which the virus gives rise is itself termed, with equal blandness, COVID-19, which refers to 'coronavirus disease 2019'.

These are uninspiring monikers – and deliberately so. Medical history is littered with examples of disease names that inadvertently insult or stigmatise people, places or animals. Examples include gay-related immune deficiency (the name first given to AIDS), Spanish flu, West Nile fever, monkeypox and swine flu. In 2015, the WHO issued recommendations that from now on diseases should be named in neutral, generic terms in order to minimise the risk of misconstruing a disease's nature or origins, or of stoking fear and racial tensions.

People write their own lexical rulebooks however. In 2020, whenever a person, newspaper or doctor uses the shorthand 'coronavirus' or 'Covid', no one imagines for a moment they are referring to the benign end of the coronavirus spectrum – the nondescript, forgettable pathogens that cause banal diseases like the common cold. In this book, I have chosen to mimic the vocabulary we tend to use colloquially in the hospital –'coronavirus' and 'Covid'.

The WHO's linguistic intervention matters. Earlier informal names for the new disease – Wuhan virus, Chinese flu – trigger a wave of ugliness and overt xenophobia towards East Asian individuals and communities. Despite this, the US president, Donald Trump, will persist in using the inflammatory moniker 'Chinese flu' all the way into the autumn of the 2020 presidential elections.

In early February, police forces in London, Newcastle, Sheffield, Manchester, York, Portsmouth and Southampton report investigating multiple incidents of verbal and physical abuse towards members of the Chinese community. A young woman celebrating her birthday in Birmingham is beaten unconscious after defending a Chinese friend from abuse. The victim, twenty-nine-year-old Meera Solanki, describes being attacked in a bar after confronting the man who told her friend to 'take your fucking coronavirus and take it back home'. Meanwhile, the University of Southampton's Chinese Students and Scholars Association feels compelled to create an anti-racism poster with the words: 'I am not a virus. I am a human.'

One day towards the middle of February my daughter, Abbey, who is nine years old, comes home from school in tears. Such is her distress, it takes a while to coax from her an explanation. It turns out that the worlds of the Black Death and SARS-CoV-2 – which were, for me, so irreconcilable – have collided in her classroom, where grisly rumours are spreading like wildfire. A 'Chinese plague' has arrived in the UK, she tells me, killing everyone who catches it within a week. 'I don't want to get buboes,' she sobs. 'I don't want to die.' Her only reference point for a plague is the last major epidemic of the bubonic plague to occur in Britain – the Great Plague that preceded the Great Fire of London, killing a quarter of the city's population in eighteen months. What had captivated the children as a topic of primary school history is now vividly, horribly close to home.

After explaining in child-centred terms why coronavirus is a much less alarming prospect, I try to explore with Abbey how the phrase 'Chinese plague' might make her Chinese friends at school feel. It all seems to go well, and I allow myself a brief moment of parental smugness until, the next morning, she runs off at full tilt towards the playground yelling gleefully, 'Who wants to know about the cranna plague?'

*

Six weeks after he arrived at the hospice, ostensibly in the last short days of his life, Steve, my patient with motor neurone disease, continues to defy his doctors' expectations. The nurses now suction the secretions from his mouth and throat, enabling Tessa to re-inhabit the role of his wife without the burden of knowing that his survival – his very ability to breathe – hinges on herself and her suctioning skills. Several times already he has suddenly stopped breathing and only the emergency actions of his nursing team – hauling him upright, slapping his back, suctioning phlegm, *come on, Steve* – have triggered another shuddering inhalation.

'It's a relief to know he's here,' Tessa confesses one day. I stare into her weary eyes and wonder briefly at the nature of sacrifice, at what we will give of ourselves, without hesitation, to another whom we love. For the last six months of her life – from the moment her husband received his terminal diagnosis – Tessa has devoted all she has to him. Every hospital appointment, every scan, every procedure, all the losses and diminishments as Steve's disease has marched on – Tessa has been at his side for them all. Suctioning, cleaning, wiping, feeding, coordinating the medications and the therapies and the equipment and the speaking aids. No carers at home to help shoulder the load. Just Tessa, alone, determined to give her husband what he needs, irrespective of personal cost.

'Tessa, I don't think there are many people who would have been able to do what you have done,' I say. 'You've been a wife, nurse, carer, physio, counsellor, mother, dietician, pharmacist. Steve has only been able to stay at home as long as he did because you've managed to achieve something extraordinary – and I really want you to know that.'

Her face quivers a little and I glance away. I do not imagine praise is something she has heard very often since Steve's diagnosis and the last thing I want to do is embarrass her. And yet, like thousands of other invisible carers all over the country, she has conducted her work of caring remarkably, unstintingly – these unsung labours of love and duty that put the rest of us to shame.

'Sometimes I wish it was over,' she admits, 'because I find it so painful to see how he suffers, what it does to him. But he wants to live, he's never stopped wanting to live.'

Steve's body clings to life and will not let go. He can scarcely breathe or swallow unaided. His heart has already stopped once. And yet his flesh, like his mind, is sinewy strong, every fibre bent on endurance.

Together, we talk about what is to come. Tessa wavers between tears and steel. She is resolved to be whatever Steve needs, all the way to the end. And, as so often at work, I am struck anew by the extraordinariness of so-called ordinary people, by the resilience and decency that lurk in our spines, awaiting these occasions of titanic calibration. People measure up so reliably, so remarkably, and bearing witness is my privilege.

February half term week is chaotic and violent. One of the most intense cyclones ever recorded outside the tropics leaves much of Europe battered and drowned beneath rainstorms. Severe flooding and the deaths of several citizens dominate the front pages. Amid the immediate tumult – winds so ferocious they whip the air from your lungs, deluges of Biblical proportions – it is easy to overlook, at least to begin with, the tempest of another kind brewing in northern Italy, favoured destination for half-term school ski trips.

It starts, as storms do, with the faintest of gusts, the merest suggestion of violence. A case of Covid is documented in Lombardy, Italy's most populous and wealthiest region. Hardly a surprise in a population of 10 million people. But two days later, on 21 February, the cases in Lombardy have leapt to 16 and one patient has died. Fast forward another four days and the death toll is now 11, with 322 cases documented. By 3 March, there will be 79 deaths and over a thousand cases recorded. In real time, the inhabitants of Lombardy have become the living, breathing, expiring illustration of the meaning of the word 'exponential'.

In his book *How Contagion Works*, written mid-pandemic, the Italian physicist and author Paolo Giordano applies his cool scientist's eye to the vertiginous spectacle of numbers in Italy catapulting out of control. Of the unfolding catastrophe in Lombardy, he writes: 'It's not what we want to hear and – crucially – it's not what we are programmed to expect. Mathematically speaking, we expect growth to be linear. We can't help it.'

Giordano's point is that Lombardy now, just like Wuhan before it, is mercilessly governed by pandemic mathematics. Suppose there are ten new cases of an infection, taking the total that day from ten to twenty. We tend to assume the same pattern will continue, so thirty the next day, forty thereafter. Instead, in an outbreak of an infectious disease, not only does the number of cases increase, but so too – entirely predictably – does the *rate* of increase itself. Two becomes four becomes eight becomes sixteen becomes thirty-two becomes sixty-four – and so on, an explosive rate of expansion.

'The actual rate of increase gets higher by the hour; it seems to be spiralling out of control,' writes Giordano. 'We could claim this was another way in which the virus caught us unaware, but it would be giving it too much credit: in reality, nature itself doesn't follow a linear structure. Nature prefers growth that is either vertigo-inducing or decidedly softer: exponentials and logarithms appear everywhere in its equations. Nature is, by its own nature, non-linear.'

For my own family, the events in northern Italy have particular significance. After his recent trips to China, Dave has been flying back and forth to Lombardy, a coincidence whose potential consequences I have made great efforts not to dwell on. But abruptly, one day in mid-February, I have no choice. I wake up before dawn drenched in sweat, feeling dreadful. Not the sore throat and congestion of a common cold, but a blistering fever and a cough that will not go away. Dave feels my forehead and brings paracetamol.

'There's no way you are well enough to go to work today,' he tells me.

'I have to go to work,' I croak. 'We're already short of doctors. If I don't turn up it will be a disaster.'

For the last ten years, Dave has borne the brunt of the almost pathological presenteeism I share with most NHS staff. This well-meaning yet misguided sense of duty – the conviction that by calling in sick we are throwing our patients to the wolves – causes sorry specimens to shiver and snuffle their way through the hospital, trailing their germs in their wake. This time, Dave has had enough.

'You're really burning up,' he insists. 'If you so much as think of going in, I will call your boss myself.'

I spend the next few days in bed, scarcely strong enough

to move. When I finally make it downstairs, I discover that the effort of getting back up again leaves me gasping for air, as though my lungs have shrivelled to nothing. For the first time, I feel afraid. Until then, I could dismiss my malaise as an unusually bad cold or perhaps, at worst, a dose of seasonal flu, but neither of those should cause this degree of breathlessness. Despite my husband's lack of symptoms, I start to wonder if his travel to China and Lombardy has indeed exposed him to infection with the novel coronavirus which, as an asymptomatic carrier, he has transmitted onwards to me.

While I am absent from the hospice, Steve begins to deteriorate. The episodes during which he cannot take another breath become more frequent and ever more frightening; each time, he presses the red emergency button that never leaves his palm. The nurses run to Steve's aid, suctioning his airway, helping him sit upright, as per his undiminished desire to live. Tessa cannot count the times she has stood in the room, an impotent onlooker, witnessing her husband reaching the brink, yet being dragged back before he topples. He insists though. He wants to keep living. No one knows more clearly than him that soon these attempts to keep him alive will fail.

One day, Steve looks more exhausted than usual. He consents to a low dose of a sedative to help take the edge off his fear. It is Valentine's Day – always bittersweet in a hospice – and both Tessa and their son, James, are there. In between episodes of gasping for breath, and to the delight and astonishment of his nurses, Steve insists on having a shave and a haircut. For a while, he seems more relaxed. Then, once more, his breathing falters.

Steve manages to turn to his son and say, 'I love you'. James kisses his father on his forehead and replies, 'I love you too, Dad'. Steve's head remains bowed and Tessa, beginning to fear the worst, reaches for the emergency buzzer. 'Dad, Dad, are you OK?' asks James. By the time the nurses rush into Steve's room, he is cradled limply in his son's arms.

Enclosed in the embrace of the two people he loves most, Steve's face begins to slacken. James picks up his phone and begins to read aloud words he has written to celebrate his father. He wants Dad to hear how much he is loved and cherished, even as he slips into unconsciousness. It is eerily calm, an almost voluntary ending, as though Steve has somehow himself dictated its timing. This is, in fact, a typical death for a patient with motor neurone disease, so much gentler than many patients fear. Steve's final breath lingers on into the silence as realisation, for his family, slowly dawns.

Later that evening, Tessa and James return to their house from the hospice. In the deadening flatness of their grief, they step through the front door into the warm embrace of the rest of their family. When Tessa is handed twelve red roses, she blinks in confusion. They were ordered weeks ago by Steve, who had looked forward to surprising his wife on Valentine's Day.

Nearly a week after the onset of my symptoms, I am sufficiently concerned about the prospect of infecting my patients on my return to work – those in a hospice being exceptionally vulnerable – that I endeavour to be tested for Covid. The 111 call centre worker I speak to is clear, however: 'You don't meet the criteria for testing.'

'I know,' I respond, fully aware that the only people eligible for tests currently are those who have been to Wuhan or Lombardy themselves and are also symptomatic. 'But I'm a doctor working in a hospice. My patients couldn't be frailer. I have a husband who *has* been to all those places and I have all the symptoms of infection myself.'

Again: 'You don't meet the criteria.'

'Look,' I try again, 'this isn't for me. It's to make sure I don't walk back into my hospice as patient zero and infect all the patients I'm trying to look after. Can't I be tested to make sure that doesn't happen? Covid would literally kill my patients.'

My efforts at negotiation cut no ice. The rules are the rules and I do not meet the criteria. No one will waste a test on me. Two weeks after first becoming ill, I am sufficiently strong to return to work, though the cough takes another month to clear. Every time I start to cough at work I apologise profusely.

'Don't worry,' I hastily say to the nurses. 'It's not a new cough, just an old one, nothing to worry about.'

But I am worried. I'm worried sick. By the end of the month there may be only 23 documented cases of the virus in Britain, yet the death toll in Italy is hurtling upwards. And, unbeknown to the public, on 26 February one of the country's foremost epidemiologists, Professor John Edmunds, and his team from the London School of Hygiene and Tropical Medicine, present their latest modelling on coronavirus at a government committee that feeds directly into SAGE – the Scientific Advisory Group for Emergencies – which itself directly advises the government. The findings are grim. If no action is taken to reduce infection rates, Edmunds has calculated, then 27 million Britons may be infected, with a predicted death toll of 380,000 people.

3

Worst-Case Scenarios

We doctors were making up to sixty calls a day. Several of us were knocked out, one of the younger of us died, others caught the thing, and we hadn't a thing that was effective in checking that potent poison that was sweeping the world.

WILLIAM CARLOS WILLIAMS,
The Autobiography of William Carlos Williams

It really should not have taken a pandemic for me to pay proper attention to the name 'virus' and its intimate connection to 'virulence'. Both, I now know, stem from the Latin word *virus*, meaning poison, venom or noxious liquid. The modern usage was coined in 1898 by the Dutch microbiologist Martinus Beijerinck to denote an infectious agent that was not a bacterium.

Then, as now, viruses are striking not so much for what they are as for what they are not. Viruses have no energy source. They cannot reproduce unaided. They are unimaginably small. The most abundant life form on Earth – there

51

are more viruses in the world than all the other forms of life added together – is so primitive that, in the opinion of most biologists, it does not qualify as a living organism at all. And yet these liminal specks, not quite living, not quite dead, 'have invaded every niche occupied by living things, including the most inhospitable places like hydrothermal vents, under the polar ice caps, and in salt marshes and acid lakes', writes Dorothy Crawford, Professor of Microbiology at the University of Edinburgh.

We are taught at school to think of cells as small; the average human body, for example, is composed of 37 trillion of them. This helps put bacteria into perspective. Each bacterium is a single-celled organism. Ten thousand of them would comfortably fit on a single grain of sand. But viruses make bacteria look like giants. The volume of a virus is around a million times smaller than that of a bacterium. So tiny are these most enigmatic of microbes that they remained invisible to the human eye until the invention of the electron microscope in the 1930s.

The crucial difference between viruses and bacteria is that, provided conditions are sufficiently damp and warm, bacteria can multiply and reproduce independently. Viruses, on the other hand, are inert and lifeless – mere inanimate particles – unless they find and invade another living organism. A virus, in short, is a parasite, its survival intimately entwined with that of its involuntary host.

Human beings are compulsive storytellers. We cannot resist imagining our lives as a dramatic and often moral struggle against macroscopic and microscopic enemies alike. Currently, the novel coronavirus is being characterised everywhere as a malicious agent, a ruthless foe, something devious, cunning and stealthy. Yet the truth is, just like any other natural organism, the virus is supremely indifferent. It doesn't 'care' about anyone or anything. It simply does what it does, innately and dumbly. Its two cardinal acts – surviving and reproducing – have nothing noble or evil about them. From the perspective of its main protagonist then, this pandemic has no plot, no motive, no narrative arc whatsoever. The new coronavirus is a mere scrap of protein and genetic material, mindlessly replicating its way through the world.

Like all micro-organisms, the coronavirus enters a human body with only one impulse: to make as many copies of itself as possible. To stand a chance of spreading, it needs to coerce human cells into churning out those copies so quickly they can dodge the body's immune system for long enough to be transmitted into another human host. The moment of entrance itself is almost certainly unmemorable. Perhaps someone close to you coughs or speaks, their exhaled breath abounding with viral particles. Now you inhale in turn, sweeping those particles through your nasal passages or down your throat into your lungs. Or maybe, instead, your hand pushes open a door where someone else, a few hours earlier, left an invisible trace of the virus. Now you absent-mindedly brush your face with your fingertips, conveying the virus to your mouth or nose. The tiniest gestures – mere butterfly wingbeats in the clamour of a day – and your fate may just have been sealed.

Coronaviruses are named after the crowns they resemble. Spikes of protein protrude from a sphere containing the viral particle's genetic material. These spikes can latch on to receptors on the surface of human cells. If the spike fits the receptor then, as neatly as a key being turned in a lock, the cell wall is breached to allow the virus inside. The coronavirus genome is composed of RNA, a close cousin of DNA, which instructs the human cell to start building and assembling new copies of the virus. Obliviously – for human cells are dumb too – the cell now functions as a coronavirus assembly line. This is an evolutionary hijacking.

The behaviour of the viral offspring precisely mimics that of their parents. They pour out of the original host cell to latch on to and infect new ones, which in turn will be transformed into hapless coronavirus factories. For as long as the pace of production of new viral particles outstrips the immune system's ability to find and destroy them, the human host will remain infected. Death is not the objective. In fact, the longer the host can coexist with its viral parasite, the greater the chances of the virus being transmitted to others. In evolutionary terms, longevity of the host is a bonus.

It is no coincidence that coronavirus irritates our airways. Every cough, every splutter, every sigh, every whispered word is an opportunity for the virus to propagate more widely. The more intimate our interactions with others, the greater the proximity of human flesh to flesh, the more effectively *we* generate a viral success story. In the zero-sum game of survival of the fittest, the number of human deaths is immaterial so long as the virus can always find new hosts in which to multiply before its predecessors expire. Right now, it has 7.8 billion of us to choose from, minus the 90,000 or so currently infected.

Like many doctors in the UK I know, I'm now glued to coverage of northern Italy's unfolding death toll as it rises day by day. It is a profoundly unsettling experience, like watching Janet

Leigh checking into the motel in Hitchcock's *Psycho*, knowing the scene in the shower is looming.

Because we *do* know, don't we? We know that the Italian government hastily quarantined eleven northern towns back on 23 February in a draconian effort – by European standards – to contain the outbreak. We know that since then, the numbers of cases and deaths have soared in Lombardy. And we know how this played out a month ago far away in central China, where the death toll now stands at 3000. My stomach knots with anxiety. Earlier, a colleague messaged me: 'Lombardy's going to be the next Wuhan, isn't it?' My reply was forlorn: 'I hope not. I just really hope not.'

I keep scouring the latest coronavirus numbers online for Wuhan and Lombardy. I can't help myself. I don't know whether the data are reliable and, frankly, I hope they are not, because these figures are stopping me sleeping. A week ago, Italy had around 500 cases of coronavirus, with 12 patients having died from it. I look to see when China was at the same stage in its outbreak: back on 22 January. Then, in China, there were 571 cases and 17 deaths. A week later there were thirteen times as many cases – 7711 – and ten times as many deaths – 170. I am no epidemiologist, but it is hard not to believe Lombardy's future is ominous.

One night in early March, I turn from my smartphone to the poetry of William Carlos Williams, the great American physician and writer. I open my book at the poem 'Spring and All'. Written in 1923, its first lines astonish me:

> *By the road to the contagious hospital*
> *under the surge of the blue . . .*

Williams' subsequent description of young shoots beginning to emerge from a grim winter wasteland encapsulates the rawness and fragility of early spring: 'They enter the new world naked, / cold, uncertain of all / save that they enter.' But it is *where* this rebirth takes place – alongside the road to a hospital for infectious diseases – that takes my breath away. A few years before he wrote the poem, the hospital Williams mentions would have been filled to bursting with casualties of the deadliest pandemic in human history, the Spanish flu of 1918–20. Of the estimated 50 to 100 million lives it claimed worldwide, 650,000 were Americans.

In *Pale Rider*, her masterful account of this viral outbreak and its human cost, the historian Laura Spinney writes:

> The flu resculpted human populations more radically than anything since the Black Death. It influenced the course of the First World War and, arguably, contributed to the second. It pushed India closer to independence, South Africa closer to apartheid, and Switzerland to the brink of civil war. It ushered in universal healthcare and alternative medicine, our love of fresh air and our passion for sport.

It has never occurred to me that Williams himself might have treated patients with the Spanish flu. But the bleakness of the landscape he depicts, into which new life so wilfully thrusts itself, is surely more than mere metaphor. I reach obsessively for my phone – the insomniac's curse – and there, sure enough, in the cobalt glow in the palm of my hand, I find Williams describing how he cared for Spanish flu victims. 'They'd be sick one day and gone the next,' he writes bluntly in his autobiography. 'Just like that, fill up and die.'

I read on. A century divides me from this doctor in New Jersey. In the absence of protective equipment, vaccines and treatments – nothing whatsoever with which to fight the potent poison – Williams treats patients with influenza regardless. Even his belief that he has become infected himself does not dampen his sense of clinical duty: 'One day I thought I would be the next. I figured I'd work until noon then quit and hit the pallet. I took some aspirin, worked like mad to finish my list, and at noon it was over. I felt tip top and kept on working.'

My mind turns to the doctors and nurses in the hospitals of Lombardy who, like Williams, will be working round the clock, resolutely helping their patients. I realise that of the many millions of victims of the Spanish flu, I have no idea how many were healthcare professionals.

On the morning of 3 March, I discover quite how much – unusually for me – I have been yearning for authority. To my immense relief, the Prime Minister gives his first televised press conference on coronavirus, flanked by the government's Chief Medical Officer, Chris Whitty, and the Chief Scientific Adviser, Patrick Vallance. Each adviser is not only a doctor, he is a former professor of medicine with impeccable academic credentials. Whitty, to my delight, was even, in his former life, an epidemiologist. Finally – urged on, I presume, by events in Lombardy – the government appears to be taking coronavirus seriously.

The publication of the UK's twenty-eight-page Coronavirus Action Plan is the reason behind today's press conference. In a Downing Street hall with man-sized Union Jacks behind the podium, the assembled journalists are treated – if that is the right word – to some sober, measured, scientific analysis. I have a day of annual leave and watch every word live from my sofa. The longer Whitty and Vallance talk, the less crushing the weight on my shoulders feels.

'Central to all of this is making sure that we protect the vulnerable,' says Vallance in his opening statement to the press. 'The highest-risk groups are the elderly and those with pre-existing illnesses, and those are the ones we've got to take most care to protect during this.'

It's everything I want to hear, everything I want to believe is happening. For the first time since I learned of the death of the Chinese ophthalmologist Li Wenliang, I feel the pandemic – at least locally – is in safe hands. The entire UK population is being treated, en masse, to two eminent doctors' best bedside manner – and how the country has been aching for it. I can relax, I believe. Someone else has got this. Smarter, wiser, far more experienced doctors than me. It is going to be OK now.

At one point in the press conference, my relief briefly falters. Boris Johnson, in replying to a journalist's question, reassures him that everything will be fine because 'We have a fantastic health service and it is well capable of handling the most tremendous pressures, as everyone knows.'

I cannot help but wince at this. We are indeed depressingly familiar with the pressures under which the NHS delivers care. But these induce endemic weakness, not resilience. Such is the mismatch between NHS resources and the needs of patients, we can scarcely provide a fit-for-purpose service in summer. The added stresses of winter and seasonal flu are enough to tip us annually into full-blown crisis. Patients on trolleys lining hospital corridors are now grimly iconic of an NHS pared to the bone. And this is categorically *not* a sign of NHS robustness. Quite the opposite. How can a health service so stripped of spare capacity cope with the demands of a once-in-a-lifetime global pandemic? I bite my lip and think longingly of Germany's twenty-nine intensive care beds per 100,000 people – four times the number of ICU beds in Britain.

It gets worse. The Channel 4 News health and social care editor, Victoria Macdonald, asks the Prime Minister if he has yet to develop his own personal policy on shaking hands. Johnson's reply is so startling I think I must have misunderstood it. 'I'm shaking hands continuously,' he answers, smiling broadly. 'I was at a hospital the other night where I think there were a few coronavirus patients and I shook hands with everybody, you will be pleased to know, and I continue to shake hands.'

My expletives are violent and unrepeatable. I'm distraught that this opening salvo in a major public health campaign has just been undermined by the man purporting to lead it. Is he actually unaware of what NHS staff are wearing before going near anyone suspected of having coronavirus? Have the photos splashed all over the front pages – those doctors decked out in such extravagant PPE they look like astronauts from a sci-fi B-movie – somehow passed the Prime Minister by? In ten seconds, Johnson has torpedoed the efforts of his scientific advisers to appraise us of the gravity of the situation. Apparently, all you need to face down coronavirus is a bit of oomph and bravado. No need to overreact, folks.

My phone burns all day with my colleagues' incredulity. Our WhatsApp groups are not for the faint-hearted. Our disbelief is underpinned by hard medicine. Every public health intervention, every effort to persuade a population to behave in ways that promote their own health and wellbeing, hinges fundamentally on trust and clarity. But this is never truer than during a pandemic, when a species' *behaviour* as much as its biology determines the numbers in which it will be felled by a microbe.

As things stand, just like for William Carlos Williams a century ago, we have no treatments for this virus and no vaccines to prevent people from catching it. High-tech modern medicine may be able to transplant faces, build bionic eyes and genetically engineer cures for cancer, yet all we have to keep coronavirus at bay is handwashing, wearing masks and keeping our distance from each other. The very last thing we need from our political leaders, therefore, is ambiguity or inconsistency about how much these measures matter. A population's best defence against a pandemic is *itself*: the public acting collectively in ways that outwit its microscopic invader.

All of this has just been highlighted to the government in the starkest terms. The day before the Prime Minister's press conference, SPI-M, the scientific committee more usually responsible for modelling the impact of influenza outbreaks, presented its latest coronavirus predictions. 'It is highly likely that there is sustained transmission of Covid-19 in the UK at present,' the report stated, before warning that if 'stringent measures' were not imposed, 80 per cent of the population was likely to become infected. According to SPI-M's best estimates of virus mortality (a case fatality rate of between 0.5 and 1 per cent), this would equate to a UK death toll of between 250,000 and 500,000 people. Social distancing has never mattered more.

Several hours after the Downing Street press conference, news emerges from Italy of the latest number of coronavirus victims there. Seventy-nine Italians have now died from the disease, nearly all of them in Lombardy. Two days later, the death toll rises to 230, a three-fold increase in only forty-eight hours.

I cannot shake my sense of dread. A few days ago, stock markets crashed worldwide, with nearly 1200 points being wiped off Wall Street's Dow Jones Index in twenty-four hours. The French president, Emmanuel Macron, warned the population that a domestic epidemic was on its way. The WHO announced that for the first time the number of new cases of coronavirus in China had been overtaken by those in the rest of the world. Countries across the globe, including Estonia, Denmark, Pakistan, Georgia, Norway, North Macedonia, Greece and Romania, are announcing their first cases of infection. And Italy and France – wisely, it seems to me – have just decided to take the drastic measure of cancelling all gatherings over 5000 people, with the Paris half marathon hastily abandoned.

I have become addicted to the Johns Hopkins University coronavirus dashboard. Here, to the best of their knowledge, the Hopkins epidemiologists post the latest daily figures for cases and deaths worldwide. The centrepiece is a dark grey map of the world on which areas of infection are depicted in circles of scarlet. Bloodstains were not, I'm sure, the desired intention, but visually the map invokes an increasingly messy, spattered, global crime scene: the entire world in the act of being daubed in blood.

My husband starts telling me to put my phone away. 'Stop reading about it,' Dave urges. 'What's the point in speculating about worst-case scenarios?'

'But Dave, it's *already* a worst-case scenario. You should read what the doctors and nurses are saying in Lombardy.'

'No, Rach, I definitely should not. And you shouldn't either.'

I hesitate, the wife in me at odds with the doctor. Our marriage is constructed on truthfulness. False reassurance feels perilously close to lying. Yet the judicious framing and reframing of risk to others is an essential skill in medicine. Doctors must know when to be blunt and when to forbear, to seed knowledge and understanding at a depth and a pace that avoid bludgeoning all hope from a patient. Above all, this delicate balance of circumspection with candour must proceed on a patient's terms, not those of their doctor. It's a high-wire walk that often demands all my expertise, and it is certainly not one I wish to undertake with my husband. So, I try to conceal my anxiety from this point onwards. As dishonesty goes, it's benign and well meaning. Still, I feel uneasy. It goes against the grain of our marriage.

By the end of the first week of March, events in northern Italy are somehow both unimaginable yet filling our screens. There are interviews with stunned Italians who have just watched their elderly parents being loaded into ambulances, never to see them again. Doctors and nurses are speaking out in desperation on social media, appalled at the horror unfolding inside their hospitals and hoping to persuade more of the public to stay inside.

'The message of the danger of what is happening is not reaching people,' says Dr Daniele Macchini in a post shared thousands of times on Facebook. A doctor at the Humanitas Gavazzeni Hospital in overwhelmed Bergamo, he describes his hospital's frantic attempts to prepare in advance for the outbreak: 'All this rapid transformation brought in the corridors of the hospital an atmosphere of surreal silence and emptiness that we still did not understand, waiting for a war that was yet to begin and that many (including me) were not so sure would ever come with such ferocity.' With the 'tsunami' having arrived, he continues: 'The situation is now nothing short of dramatic. No other words come to mind. The war has literally exploded and the battles are uninterrupted day and night.'

This cannot, surely, be what is to come in our hospitals?

'One after the other the departments that had been emptied are filling up at an impressive rate,' the Italian doctor writes. 'The cases multiply, we arrive at the rate of 15–20 hospitalisations a day all for the same reason. The results of the swabs now come one after the other: positive, positive, positive. Suddenly the emergency room is collapsing.'

Such is the volume of severely ill patients now arriving at the doors of Lombardy's hospitals that A&E departments, operating theatres and recovery areas have all been turned into impromptu intensive care units, and additional ventilators – machines that mechanically breathe for patients whose lungs have failed – are being rushed in from every corner of Italy. But still the patients keep coming. As the doctors and nurses themselves fall ill, those still standing are forced to work ever more gruelling hours. Before long, they find they are connecting their own colleagues to the ventilators that may or may not save their lives.

Just as the late Li Wenliang became iconic of doctors' bravery in China, so too does the image of a nurse from Cremona, Elena Pagliarini, become a visual symbol of Italy's furious struggle against coronavirus. The small Lombardy town is more usually revered for its musical heritage, with Stradivarius among its most renowned violin makers. Now, a photo of

Pagliarini at work, slumped unconscious over her desk still wearing her gloves, masks, scrubs and gown, is shared around the world. So exhausting were the preceding ten hours in which she endeavoured to keep her patients alive, she fell asleep the moment she sat down.

Perhaps the most chilling news of all from Lombardy is that some hospitals are having to resort to a form of rationing more suited to battlefields than modern health services, denying some patients intensive care beds not because they are beyond saving but because the supply of beds has run dry. The *Times* newspaper reports that ordinarily Lombardy has only 750 intensive care beds, yet between 2700 and 3200 are predicted to be needed in the region by the end of March – and doctors and nurses are dropping like flies. Such is the severity of the bed crisis, the Italian Society of Anaesthesia Analgesia Resuscitation and Intensive Care (SIAARTI) resorts to publishing fifteen ethical recommendations to help doctors decide who is allocated – or denied – an ICU bed. 'We do not want to discriminate,' said Dr Luigi Riccioni, co-author of the new guidance on how to prioritise treatment of coronavirus cases in hospitals. The aim, he explains, is to ensure individual medical staff are not left alone 'in front of such a difficult ethical choice'.

Meanwhile, the slew of bodies requiring cremation and burial is quickly becoming unmanageable. Local funeral directors, many of whom are now sick themselves, simply cannot cope with demand. In the cool darkness of Lombardy's cavernous churches – a kind of dignity, I suppose, amid the turmoil outside – growing numbers of coffins now lie stacked and silent, each concealing a body awaiting interment. The belongings of the deceased are sealed inside plastic bags placed on the flagstones beside them. Grieving family members are barred from retrieving them for their own protection. Italy's military police are summoned. Officers load army trucks with piles of coffins to distribute to any crematorium in the country with spare capacity. Once more, I cannot help but think back to my primary school days. None of this feels far away at all from the time of the Black Death when the nameless dead were transported in horse-drawn carts to mass burials and improvised plague pits.

In a little over a fortnight, Italians will discover that coronavirus has claimed the lives of 13,000 of their fellow citizens. The country is in the grip of a humanitarian catastrophe.

4

A Brilliant Plan

What's the bravest thing you ever did?
He spat in the road a bloody phlegm.
Getting up this morning, he said.

CORMAC MCCARTHY, *The Road*

'Hello, John. How are you feeling today?'

'Well now, just have a look out of the window,' he replies, beckoning me over. 'See that? Look, up on the tree over there. See? Look!'

I squint through the glass, trying to spot what has animated him. There. A woodpecker is shimmying up and down the trunk, occasionally flashing its scarlet rump like a can-can girl flaunting her bloomers. I cannot help but smile. Delight, just like fear, is contagious.

John Forrest arrived in the hospice a fortnight ago with one of the most sluggish of malignancies, a skin cancer known as a squamous cell carcinoma. It typically appears on sun-exposed areas, in John's case the right side of his forehead. The merest blemish at first, it advanced so surreptitiously he scarcely noticed it was there. Months and then years went by. John was, after all, a man in his seventies and appropriately gnarled for a former farm labourer. One imperfection rolled into another until his face was as furrowed and flecked as the land he'd worked for decades. By the time this particular defect stood out from the rest, it had begun to work its way inwards, embedding itself within the nerves and bones of his head and neck. Despite a series of increasingly desperate surgeries – 'heroic' is the term some surgeons still reach for – the cancer resisted all attempts at excision.

Today, John's ability to savour small joys is a wonder all of its own. The cancer has assaulted his face so systematically it is hard to believe there can be any scope for pleasure. One empty eye socket – the eyeball long gone – has been nibbled and gnawed into a crater so deep that bare bone is on permanent display. From a certain angle, tongue and teeth are visible. Tumour has torn down and rebuilt a face of sorts, but one that bulges, collapses, gapes and billows, its architecture barely recognisable as human.

None of this seems to dampen John's capacity for living. His speech is impaired, his pain sometimes severe, yet the blackbirds, blue skies and woodpeckers in the hospice gardens never go unnoticed. He knows every one of the nurses' names and how to make them smile. Despite being almost unable to swallow, he takes his few sips of Guinness every evening with a reverence that borders on devotional. He is used to pulses of horror distorting his visitors' faces before they manage to get a grip on their features. He responds with patience and magnanimity.

'I know what I look like,' he once told me. 'I'd be scared too, if I wasn't so used to it.'

There is no one for John back at home. He never married and his only living relatives are both emotionally and geographically distant. Something of a loner, I imagine, he now seems to relish every chance to impart his knowledge of nature to his carers. With his one eye, he studies the woodpecker contentedly.

'It's a greater spotted, not the lesser,' he tells me. 'Much more common, bigger too. The little one's not much bigger than a sparrow, you know.'

We share a moment watching it jig across the bark, a dapper prospector of beetles. Unlike John, I have half my mind on what will come next, a conversation I wish could be avoided. The horrors of what is unfolding in Italy still feel light years away from the depths of rural Oxfordshire. But like everyone in the NHS, we fear what is coming and we know we must prepare. Every day now the news is bleaker. The death toll in Britain has recently surged from zero to over 300 and in Italy 6000 people have already lost their lives to coronavirus. Among the hospice staff, rumours are rife. 'What about PPE? Will we have coronavirus patients here? Is it true patients have already died in the John Radcliffe? Have you heard that doctors are dying in Lombardy?' None of us have any answers. It feels dizzying, vertiginous, to know so little, like being walked to a ledge in a blindfold.

Amid all the whispers and uncertainty, I find relief in focusing on a tangible task that, though painful, puts patients first. The hospice doctors are asking our inpatients, one by one, what their wishes would be if they became infected with coronavirus.

'There's something I need to have a chat with you about, John,' I begin, choosing my words with care. 'Have you been following the news about coronavirus?'

He grimaces in response. 'Awful. I hope they find a vaccine soon.'

I nod in agreement. 'We're having to think ahead about something important, which is what happens if patients here catch the virus. That's what I want to ask you about, John. I need to know your views on that. There's no reason why you should catch it, but if you did, do you have a sense of whether you would want to go to hospital to be treated or stay here with us?'

To my surprise, John smiles without hesitation. 'No hospital for me, Rachel. I know I don't have long. I'd like to stay here if I can. But − now, this is important − if it's better for the other patients for me to go to hospital, then you send me in. I wouldn't want anyone else to catch it because of me, so you send me in if you're worried about that.'

For a moment, his smile wavers. These are matters, we both know, of deadly seriousness. I have just asked a man already close to death to recalibrate his wishes around dying. In the event of his infection with coronavirus, a hospital admission might offer him a long shot at a few more weeks of life, while remaining in the hospice could bring death prematurely. Yet none of these mortal permutations interest him. His immediate instinct − his only impulse − is to consider the impact of his wishes on others. What matters to him is ensuring he does not endanger the other patients in the hospice. It catches my breath in my throat, the generosity − the selflessness − of someone like John who has lost so much, whose life is at its end, and yet chooses to give, to keep on giving to others. It is easy to forget, amid the frenetic business of living, that most people try to be good.

'That's incredibly decent of you, John,' I say, 'to put the others first.'

He shakes his head. I can see he thinks I'm talking nonsense or wishes, at least, for us to collude in that judgement. The last thing I wish to do is embarrass him. We sit for a while in easy silence by the window, watching the tireless excavations of the greater spotted woodpecker.

That night, I turn John's words over and over. I never foresaw that my job would one day entail walking from bedside to bedside, negotiating with each of my patients in turn where they would hope to be treated if struck down by a pandemic. This is field medicine, basically. A form of hard-nosed rationality born out of necessity. We are having to respond to unimagined times and the wrongness of it goes beyond unease: it is painfully visceral.

'I don't think it's right that we're doing this. It's not fair on the patients,' one of the nurses said to me earlier. Her concern stemmed entirely from compassion. Forcing a wardful of patients with terminal illnesses to consider dying even more prematurely from coronavirus cannot, in any sense, be construed as kind. But it is, I would argue, respectful. *Not* having the conversations may avoid a degree of distress, but at the cost of denying our patients their agency. Should the hospice become infected, and the patients themselves too unwell to express their wishes, we need to know we are not considering interventions or treatments that run against what has never been voiced. To my relief, all our patients elect to remain with us if infected. It is hard to imagine someone as battered by disease as a typical hospice patient surviving the onslaught of coronavirus – and what is occurring in some British hospitals now is nothing short of hellish.

By mid-March, everything has changed. What was once a distant threat, a looming menace, has arrived in Britain and is behaving exactly as feared. I am hearing terrible things from my colleagues in London, whose wards are filling with cases. A friend takes to social media in sheer desperation. Distraught at the complacency with which the population is clearly at large on the streets, living life as enthusiastically and sociably as normal, Julia Prague tweets: 'As a frontline doctor in London – you really, really need to take this seriously – it is bad – it is really bad – already – and it's predicted to be worse by next weekend – too many people really don't get it yet – stay indoors!! Seriously!'

Another junior doctor in intensive care shares an impromptu selfie on Twitter one evening. Her hair is matted with sweat, cheeks etched with pressure damage from her face mask and eyes bloodshot with exhaustion. Like Julia, Natalie Silvey's aim is to jolt people into greater vigilance. Her tweet reads: 'This is the face of someone who just spent 9 hours in personal protective equipment moving critically ill Covid-19 patients around London. I feel broken – and we are only at the start. I am begging people, please please do social distancing and self isolation.'

Nat had volunteered, alongside her consultant, to spend the day transporting London's most perilously unwell patients to the units with the best chance of saving their lives. I am used to seeing her impeccably made up and beaming from her online selfies. But now, in a word, she looks shell-shocked. You want to scoop her up and hold her tight and tell her she never has to endure a day like that again. But this is only the beginning. 'Those red/purple marks across my face are from my mask and are deeper than you think,' she continues. 'Today I have seen just what Covid-19 is doing and now I just want to scream at people to listen to us.'

In no sense are these two experienced doctors prone to exclamation. They simply cannot bear what they are witnessing inside the walls of their hospitals, juxtaposed with the complacency of public behaviour outside. The tweets go viral but the behaviour continues. Why *would* people lock themselves away in self-imposed house arrest when no one in authority is insisting they do so? In times of uncertainty, we rely, do we not, on our leaders' lead? The Prime Minister has only recently chosen to spend a Saturday afternoon watching the England v. Wales Six Nations international, alongside 82,000 other rugby fans crammed into the stands at Twickenham. It generates approving headlines from some of the press – 'Boris Johnson Braves Coronavirus Outbreak with Pregnant Fiancée to Support England' in the *Daily Express*, for example – but many doctors, myself among them, are distraught at the symbolic defiance. Official medical guidance not to shake each other's hands and keep a cautious distance means nothing when the PM himself ignores it.

Three days after the Twickenham match, on 10 March, Germany announces its decision to cancel all large events over 1000 people in size. The same day in the UK, the annual Cheltenham Races begin. Over the course of the next four days a total of 250,000 people jostle and cluster together in the Cheltenham stands, cheering on their favoured horses. The decision not to cancel feels like an act of biomedical vandalism.

Throughout this period, I am in close contact with doctors for whom coronavirus is already an intimate reality. Though the disease has yet to move westwards out of London in significant numbers, we are bracing ourselves in Oxfordshire for what is to come. I am hungry for every scrap of clinical knowledge already gleaned in the capital.

'It's scary as hell how quickly patients deteriorate,' a colleague in a major London teaching hospital tells me. Not exactly what I wanted to hear. Arjun, who specialises in infectious diseases, goes on: 'They're not all old, they're not all frail. We've got people in their thirties on ICU.'

'Jesus. You mean with no co-morbidities?'

'*Yes.* None whatsoever. Young, fit, healthy. A damn sight younger than you, Rach.'

'OK, OK, no need to put me in the higher-risk bracket, thanks.'

We are laughing, because this is how medics like to defuse the tensions of practice, but the conversation is deadly serious.

'Sometimes they come in looking like death,' Arjun continues. 'We're calling ICU to review them pretty much the moment they've come through the door. But other times, they feel remarkably well with it. You can't believe how low their sats are. You do the X-ray and see the classic Covid whiteout – but the patient has no idea how sick they are. It's like we're learning on the job, patient by patient. We basically know nothing about this virus.'

Arjun is referring to an intriguing coronavirus phenomenon which doctors briefly christen, with a macabre sense of alliteration, 'happy hypoxia'. Typically, when an illness attacks the lungs and oxygen levels in the bloodstream plummet, a patient feels increasingly breathless. A healthy person usually has oxygen saturations of at least 95 per cent. Yet in some cases of infection with coronavirus, patients are found to have extraordinarily low oxygen levels – percentages in the 70s, 60s or even 50s – while feeling entirely comfortable, sat up in bed and chatting with their doctors. This mismatch between severity of disease and patient experience seems to defy basic biology. Oxygen levels as low as this would ordinarily be expected to cause not only great distress, but also unconsciousness or even death.

The peculiar response of some patients to hypoxia is an early example of how poorly we understand the ways in which the virus deranges normal human physiology. Doctors speculate that the phenomenon may be caused by coronavirus triggering abnormal blood clotting in the tiniest vessels of the lungs. But, as with so much about this novel pathogen, nobody really knows. As Arjun puts it: 'It feels like we're making it up as we go along.'

I can't shake Arjun's phrase from my head. What distinguishes a doctor from a quack or a charlatan is science – the empirical data upon which our practice is based. Should you suffer a heart attack and we reach for a particular constellation of drugs, we can do so, these days, with confidence. Randomised controlled trials have demonstrated that these medications are the ones that are most likely to increase your life expectancy. It is not that we take evidence for granted. The effort that goes into running a clinical research trial is momentous, arduous and often futile. But data defines what we do, and academic clinicians devote their lives to seeking it. Coronavirus has cut all of this clean away. There are no textbooks, no protocols, only the sketchiest of data. The disease is too new, too misunderstood. We have no idea what works yet. Across the globe, guesswork and anecdote and shared hands-on experience is all that doctors have to go on.

At 9 a.m. on 12 March – the day after the WHO officially declares a pandemic – Robert Peston, the seasoned political editor of ITV News, publishes a blog entitled 'British government wants UK to acquire coronavirus "herd immunity"'. The Johnson administration has a predilection for floating official policy announcements in advance via anonymous briefings from unnamed 'government sources'. Peston, known in Westminster circles for his impeccable Downing Street contacts, appears to have been given exclusive access to one such briefing, though the source of the information contained in his blog is not made explicit.

'The strategy of the British government in minimising the impact of Covid-19,' he writes, 'is to allow the virus to pass through the entire population so that we acquire herd immunity.' This, he explains, is 'what happens to a group of people or animals when they develop sufficient antibodies to be resistant to a disease'. Until now, if the public have heard of herd immunity at all, it is likely to have been in the context of the raging debate between proponents of vaccination (that is to say, doctors and scientists) and the ferociously vocal 'anti-vaxxer' movement comprising people who believe, against all evidence to the contrary, that vaccination does more harm than good. The phrase 'herd immunity' captures the idea that once a critical proportion of a population has been vaccinated, thus acquiring antibodies to a disease, the remainder will also be protected since enough individuals have developed immunity to prevent transmission between the vaccinated and unvaccinated alike. In a highly infectious disease such as measles, vaccination rates of 95 per cent are required to achieve strong herd immunity. Coronavirus, being less infectious, is estimated to require an infection rate of 60 per cent, meaning around 40 million Britons would need to be infected to achieve herd immunity.

The triumph of vaccination, of course, is that it controls transmission of an infectious disease *without* the population being harmed in the process. Presenting herd immunity as a strategic aim in the absence of a vaccine is an altogether different matter. It entails vast numbers of people succumbing to a disease before the population, overall, develops immunity. With an estimated 1 per cent coronavirus mortality rate, this equates to an approximate British death toll of 400,000 people.

A crucial part of the strategy, Peston elaborates, is to delay the speed of transmission until a vaccine is developed. This will ensure 'that those who suffer the most acute symptoms are able to receive the medical support they need, and such that the health service is not overwhelmed and crushed by the sheer number of cases it has to treat at any one time'. The delays will be achieved initially by simple social distancing measures in addition to increased handwashing. A new wariness about physical contact with others, working from home if possible, and keeping isolated if we develop symptoms of coronavirus. 'For what it's worth, ministers are looking with grim bemusement at the debate in football's governing bodies about banning the public from stadia,' Peston adds. 'They fear this fuels alarmism and do not think playing matches behind closed doors is necessary at this stage.'

There is, however, a crucial flaw in the strategy as outlined. If the aim of social distancing measures is only to *delay*, as opposed to *reduce*, the overall spread of coronavirus, then the death toll may remain largely unchanged, albeit not concentrated in one rapid surge that could overwhelm NHS capacity. For this is a virus with no known treatments or cure. There is no vaccine. Designing one may take eighteen months or more, despite the best efforts of scientists across the globe. Doctors' options are therefore rudimentary: essentially, we can support failing lungs with extra oxygen and minimise the risks of superimposed bacterial infections with powerful antibiotics. Even intensive care, in the end, is only a temporary holding measure, a means of supporting failing organs until – we hope – the body eventually recovers from the damage the virus has inflicted. I cannot help but fear that the government is pinning everything on an as-yet non-existent science.

That evening, Boris Johnson appears once more in Downing Street, flanked by his Chief Medical Officer, Chris Whitty, and Chief Scientific Adviser, Patrick Vallance. Gone is the Prime Minister's former bonhomie. He wears his gravity awkwardly, like an ill-fitting suit. This is the 'worst public health crisis for a generation', he tells us. 'It is going to spread further and I must level with you, the British public. Many more families are going to lose loved ones before their time.'

Johnson then announces a significant policy shift. From now on, anyone with a new continuous cough or a high temperature is advised to self-isolate at home for seven days, rather than only those individuals who have just returned from a high-risk area such as Wuhan. There is, however, I note uneasily, no movement on closing schools or banning large gatherings. The best available science does not warrant this, we are told. Nor are *any* new measures announced that are specifically tailored towards protecting vulnerable groups – namely, those aged over seventy or with pre-existing medical conditions – other than advising them not to go on cruises. Indeed, Whitty explicitly rules out recommending the self-isolation of the elderly and infirm: 'While we will need to move to that stage, we do not think this is the right moment along the pandemic to do so. But that point will come.'

The most startling moment of the press conference is when Robert Peston's blog, which I have tried all day not to fret about, appears to be formalised on live television. Whitty announces that the UK can no longer contain coronavirus – it is freely transmitting throughout the country – and we are therefore moving to the next stage of the strategy, that of merely endeavouring to delay its spread. From now on, new cases in the community will not be tracked at all. 'It is no longer necessary for us to identify every case,' he states. In future, only hospital cases will be tested for coronavirus. To me, the abandonment of efforts to trace the virus's spread feels like the tacit embrace of herd immunity – an act, essentially, of capitulation.

As the conference draws to a close, I sit slumped on the sofa feeling simultaneously nauseous and stupid. The children are laughing next door with their dad. I envy their levity, their lightness. There must be a big picture I am failing to under-stand, something to rally my spirits. These are clever, brilliant, eminent scientists. Yet their strategy, to my non-expert and undoubtedly paranoid eyes, is defeatism. It's out there, it's spreading, it can no longer be controlled – and, as of now, we are seemingly throwing in the towel, abandoning any effort to keep a track on cases. Worse – and here I think painfully of my seventy-seven-year-old mother alone in her flat – the only measure to date specifically aimed at protecting individuals like her is to dissuade them half-heartedly from setting off on cruises. Surely, in combination, those two approaches are deadly? What has happened to cocooning the most vulnerable? Instead, in Britain, we now have the perfect storm of sustained community transmission of a virus which (as the data from China has already told us) kills 8 per cent of the over-eighties, plus an elderly population still strolling around to meet it.

Again, that night, I can't sleep. I think of the patients I may, unknowingly, have already infected by bringing undetected coronavirus into the hospice. I worry that now, should any of them develop coronavirus-like symptoms, we will not even be able to access a test for them since hospices are not regarded as hospital settings. Above all, I am overwhelmed by the thought of all the dying to come and by how resigned the government appears to be to this.

The next morning, as public and media opposition to the new government stance builds, Patrick Vallance is sent out on the broadcast circuit in an effort at damage limitation. He tells BBC Radio 4: 'If you suppress something very, very hard, when you release those measures it bounces back, and it bounces back at the wrong time. Our aim is to try to reduce the peak, broaden the peak, not suppress it completely. Also, because the vast majority of people get a mild illness, to build up some kind of herd immunity so more people are immune to this disease and we reduce the transmission. At the same time, we protect those who are most vulnerable to it.'

Another reason to avoid being too restrictive too soon, Vallance explains, is that behavioural modelling suggests this may lead to 'isolation fatigue', in which people tire of prolonged restrictions and begin to flout them. When he is challenged directly on Sky News about why society is 'continuing as normal' when this risks 'an awful lot of people dying', he responds by stating simply: 'Well of course we do face the prospect, as the Prime Minister said yesterday, of an increasing number of people dying.'

The WHO could not disagree more vehemently with the UK's strategy. Even as Vallance tours the television studios, the WHO's director-general, Dr Tedros Adhanom Ghebreyesus, gives a briefing of his own. 'You can't fight a virus if you don't know where it is,' he tells journalists. 'Find, isolate, test and treat every case to break the chains of Covid transmission. Every case we find and treat limits the expansion of the disease.'

Meanwhile, despite the official government advice on crowds, the Premier League, Rugby Football Union and organisers of the London Marathon decide to take matters into their own hands. All their matches and the marathon are immediately suspended. Such is the domestic backlash against the government's inertia, the health secretary is forced to hastily publish a piece in the *Sunday Telegraph* newspaper denying that herd immunity was ever an aim. 'We have a plan, based on the expertise of world-leading scientists,' Matt Hancock writes. 'Herd immunity is not a part of it. That is a scientific concept, not a goal or a strategy.'

The same day, I speak again to Arjun, my London colleague in infectious diseases. 'What am I not understanding?' I ask. 'Why are they giving up on community testing? Please tell me there's something fundamental I'm not getting.'

'Rachel, there's a reason why the WHO pushes test, trace and isolate,' he replies bitterly. 'It's because it works. It worked with SARS, it worked with MERS, it worked with Ebola, it will work with this. You cannot get a grip on an epidemic if you don't know where the cases are. That is basic public health. There is no magic plan here. This is simply making do with the resources we have, only not being honest about it. It's politics. They don't have anything like the capacity to test everyone, so they've just given up on that and pretended they can justify it. It's a horror show.'

I hesitate, computing what this means.

'What's it been like on the ward for you this week?' I ask quietly.

Now it is Arjun's turn to pause. Then, this principled doctor I have known since medical school – someone who, in 2015, was one of 150 NHS volunteers to join Ebola response teams battling the pandemic in Sierra Leone – does something I have not known him do before. Arjun is never lost for words. In fact, as a rule it is impossible to stop him talking. But the pause turns into a sigh, and the sigh into something resembling a sob.

'They've downgraded our PPE,' he says.

I'm aware of this downgrade. In fact, for the last few days doctors have been lighting up social media with their bewilderment and fear after Public Health England abruptly issued new guidance on what protective equipment to wear at work. Until then, this comprised full-length, long-sleeved surgical gowns, visors, the most effective form of mask, and several pairs of gloves. Now, with no explanation – and for all but the most at-risk staff – the new recommendations comprise only a paper mask, one set of gloves, no eye protection, and a skimpy plastic apron that leaves the arms, upper chest, back and lower legs entirely exposed. Only those at increased risk of being exposed to 'aerosols' – the tiniest droplets a person exhales – need continue to wear the higher-level protection.

With Oxfordshire still treating only small numbers of cases, the full significance of the downgrade had not yet dawned on me. But Arjun is already riding the crest of the wave, working twelve-hour shifts, night or day, in the 'hot' zone of his London hospital. The doors of his ward are locked, the atmosphere oppressive. Inside, every one of the patients is infected with coronavirus. Already, in the hospital's ICU, there are colleagues lying intubated on ventilators. For him, and for every one of the frontline medics, nurses, paramedics and allied healthcare professionals, PPE is quite literally a matter of life and death.

'My ward,' says Arjun harshly, 'is where all the patients who have tested positive are, apart from the ones who need intensive care. All of them. I'm seeing patients who will die from this disease. One day, I was wearing full PPE, now we've been told not to bother with any of that. They've told us, "just treat it as though it's seasonal flu".'

The new UK standards are inexplicably *lower* than those recommended by the WHO and the European Union, both of whom advise mandatory eye protection and full-length surgi-cal gowns for all clinicians in proximity to suspected cases of coronavirus. 'A plastic apron doesn't cover you like a surgical gown does,' Arjun elaborates. 'I'm wearing the same set of scrubs seeing different patients all around the hospital, and my scrubs could have coronavirus on them.'

Now I understand what underlies his distress. Not, primarily, fear for his *own* safety, but the prospect of unwittingly endangering others. 'I am terrified. I'm seriously considering whether I can keep working as a doctor. I may be OK – I'm young and healthy – but I can't bear the thought of infecting other patients with a disease that could kill them. And that is the risk, without proper PPE. It's terrifying. It's indescribable. This is not seasonal flu. This is a new virus with greater mortality and we know much less about it. I cannot understand what the rationale and motives are. Have they given up? Are they just deciding to build up herd immunity by watching us die? The government has given up, hasn't it?'

I don't know how to answer. Everything I could say would sound platitudinous. Arjun cannot help himself. The words pour out. He can't sleep, he feels sick, he feels betrayed, he feels abandoned. His final observation is chilling. 'I cannot understand why they have stopped testing and contact tracing, either. Even hospital staff are being told we can't be tested if our own symptoms are mild. This is unbelievable. If we're not allowed to be tested, then how will we ever know how many other people – patients – we are infecting? Brilliant. What a brilliant plan.'

Of this time, David Hunter, Professor of Epidemiology and Medicine at the University of Oxford, will later write in the *New England Journal of Medicine*: 'Many clinicians and scientists have been pushing the panic button, but the alarm, if heard, was not acted on publicly ... Everyone is hoping that their gut instincts, the experience of other countries, and now the models are wrong. What is not in doubt is that barring a miracle, a treatment, and ultimately a vaccine, the NHS in the United Kingdom is about to experience a challenge unlike any other in its 70 years of existence.'

I arrive with two of my nursing colleagues from the hospice at the car park of our local hospital. We have come here to be trained in how to safely use our PPE. This afternoon, the mood at work, the newspaper headlines and even the heavens themselves have aligned in mutinous harmony. We squint up at the glowering sky, dark and steely with the threat of thunder, and laugh at the aptness of the weather.

The evening before, on 19 March, Boris Johnson delivered an unexpectedly jaunty press conference in which he assured an anxious nation we would 'turn the tide within the next twelve weeks' and 'send coronavirus packing in this country', as though it were some unwanted door-to-door salesman. He made the comments on the same day the number of Britons known to have died from the disease rose by 40 per cent to 144. The deaths, of course, were just getting started. The speech had felt like prime ministerial gaslighting.

'I don't know how much longer I can take it without lockdown,' Tanya murmurs as we walk towards the hospital entrance. 'I mean, have they actually decided to just ignore what's going on in Italy?'

Tanya is the glue that holds the hospice inpatient unit together. One of our senior nurses, she brings grace and integrity to the matter of leading a team through days that can, on occasion, be unimaginably harrowing. There is a decency about her that feels almost old-fashioned. You know without question that whatever the circumstances, she will endeavour to do the right thing. These are quiet qualities. They do not scream 'look at me' and they rarely earn riches or plaudits. Yet the longer I have worked as a doctor, the more clearly I have learned that their value is priceless. Trust is the lynchpin of any group, any team. Without it, relationships curdle.

Tanya frowns as she tucks a stray strand of hair behind her ear. I know precisely what underlies her anxiety. Her three sons are aged five, eight and eleven. Tom, the eldest, has asthma of such severity that already, four or five times in his young life, he has been rushed by ambulance to hospital. Tanya has witnessed the highly choreographed swoop of a paediatric crash team upon her son's little body, flawless and pale beneath the needles and wires, his ribs retracting with the strain of each breath, the fear in his eyes as they searched for her. Until now, each time he has escaped intensive care — but only just, a hair's breadth from the anaesthetist's cocktail, the tube slipped down a paralysed throat, a ventilator forcing the ebb and flow of each breath.

Tanya knows that difficult decisions are looming. Healthcare workers around the world are being forced to choose between their patients and their loved ones. If Tanya brought Covid back into her home, she could expose her son to a potentially fatal illness. He could perish because she chose to endanger him. What parent, she asks herself time and again, could possibly do that? Yet what nurse abandons her patients at precisely the time they need her most? Caring for others is ingrained in her marrow. Walking away would be a violation of all she is made of.

She lies awake most nights now, sifting through options. She keeps coming back to the same bleak scenario, the only prospect she thinks she can bear. She could continue to do her duty for her patients if she temporarily abandoned her husband and children, basing herself in a hotel near the hospice. They would, after all, still have each other, Tanya tells herself. They would still be a family in lockdown and maybe – maybe – she would be too hectic to miss them too fiercely. Maybe it wouldn't be too bad. In London, she knows, such estrangements are becoming widespread. At the taxpayer's expense, fathers, mothers, sons and daughters are now holed up in their hundreds in skyrise hotels adjacent to the capital's great hospitals – Tommy's, Imperial, King's, the Royal London. Each member of staff has chosen self-imposed quarantine above endangering the ones they love most deeply. Devoid of their usual clientele – the well-heeled tourists and sharp-suited executives – London's Hiltons, Park Plazas and InterContinentals are swelling with wan-faced armies of NHS doctors and nurses, the hotel laundries working overtime to fumigate never-ending mountains of corona-infested scrubs.

As I walk with my nursing colleagues through the hospital car park, it is eerily empty. We pass a security guard who takes one look at our faces and tells us to bloody well cheer up. We laugh, and I ask him what the mood is like in the hospital. He points up at the thunderclouds above.

'See that?' he tells us. 'That's what it feels like. It's not like London here yet. But it will be. It's coming for us. We're waiting for it to hit.'

5

A Long Deep Breath

*I am of certain convinced that the greatest heroes are those who
do their duty in the daily grind of domestic affairs whilst the
world whirls as a maddening dreidel.*

FLORENCE NIGHTINGALE

There always has to be a first time. And though intubation is
the emblematic procedure of the pandemic, this moment, this
patient, his pair of wide and roving eyes, is the hospital's first
time. Four people loom around his bed in the semi-darkness,
swathed in blue plastic, masked and gowned, disguised behind
thick Perspex visors. Normally, in an ICU, it is the patient
who becomes dehumanised. Punctured and crisscrossed by a
cat's cradle of wires and tubes, alive thanks only to the bedside machinery that hums and chugs and sucks and blows, a
Frankenstein version of a body.

Tonight, though, it is the doctors and nurses who appear less
than human. Veiled behind their protective equipment, they
hover like ghosts at the bedside, preparing nervously to act.

Breathtaking

Even in normal times, intubation is a serious business. In order to connect a patient via a tube to a ventilator, they must first be anaesthetised and then paralysed with drugs. Once the patient is unconscious and limp, the intensivist can set about the delicate business of depressing the tongue with a metal blade and steering the tube downwards, past the vocal cords and into the trachea. Few procedures in medicine have higher stakes. Losing an airway – failing to access the lungs – leaves a patient entirely helpless, immobilised on the edge of suffocation. Most doctors cannot cope with the intensity of managing airways. The pressure is too great, the requisite skills too daunting. Those that can – intensive care doctors, anaesthetists and emergency medics – earn their colleagues' utmost respect for possessing nerves of steel.

It's Sally, an intensive care nurse, who tells the patient. She takes his hand and leans in close, hating the necessity of raising her voice above the layers behind which she is barricaded. 'We're going to put you on a ventilator,' she says. 'We can give you much more oxygen that way. It's going to help your breathing.'

His eyes, above his mask, start to skitter wildly as if searching for something or someone to help him. The machinery bleeps as his blood pressure surges. Sally keeps holding his hand. Over and over, the same words to soothe, a litany she hopes may offer comfort. 'It's going to be all right. We're here for you. It's going to be all right.' But his face is white and bathed in sweat. She's convinced he can sense the uncertainty, somehow intuiting how out of their depth they are, the small team that is meant to be saving him.

A hush descends as the intensive care doctor moves into position for the intubation. They are huddled like supplicants around the bed, these four staff peering down on one patient. It is intimate to the point of claustrophobia. Even the air they share belongs to them and them alone. For the five are sealed inside a room especially designed to sequester infections, its negative pressure drawing in air from outside while clinging to its own contaminated vapours. That air, of course, reeks of invisible danger. Every surface and every one of the gowns and masks they wear will be thickly coated in particles of coronavirus. As they work, each team member is managing the fear that the person whose life they are trying to save may yet be the death of them.

You cannot get much closer than this. The doctor leans over directly above her patient's now slack and gaping mouth, decisively angling her blade downwards. An inch or two more and they could almost be kissing. Normally, she would have spent several minutes clutching a mask to her patient's face to fill their lungs with pure oxygen. It buys time. By elevating blood oxygen levels to nearly 100 per cent, it gives a margin of error – five minutes to play with – should something calamitous go wrong. But this time, the patient is already on pure oxygen. There is nowhere higher to go. Even worse, the moment she takes off his mask to commence the intubation, his oxygen saturations will plummet. She knows she has to act lightning fast.

At her signal, the mask is removed. A cacophony. Every alarm shrieking in unison. The patient's blood oxygen levels are dropping second by second. The monitor reads 80 per cent, then 75 per cent, then 70 per cent, and still the decimals flicker downwards. Even when her blade triggers a spasm of involuntary coughing, the intensivist maintains her poise. Aerosols of Covid now plaster her visor. No time to consider that now.

Sally is still gripping her patient's slack palm. *Get it in, get the bloody thing in.* Sats at 60 per cent now. Dangerously low. This is critical. In a few moments, the patient's heart will stop beating. 55 per cent. It's looking disastrous. And then, those grimly exultant two words – 'I'm in!' – and even as the tube is hooked up to the ventilator, the patient's sats are soaring upwards. The whole team collectively exhales.

Later that morning, at the end of her shift, Sally leaves the unit feeling stunned yet optimistic. She spent the rest of the night drawing up the cocktails of drugs her patient needed, managing the complex machinery of the ventilator, ensuring the infusions for sedation and to manage his blood pressure were delivered just so, with perfect precision. She tended to his bowels, his urine, his dry mouth and eyes. Gently, she administered the drops into each to ensure his corneas were protected by a film of moisture. He knew nothing of the tenderness with which she cared for him.

In normal times, pre-coronavirus times, relatives would likely have been clustered at the bedside. The patient's wife, perhaps, bearing gifts and pictures of the grandchildren. Hand-drawn cards in psychedelic felt-tipped pen declaring to the world: 'I love you, Grampy!' But now, his loved ones are entirely cut off, unable to visit for fear that by doing so, they may in turn infect others. The supreme cruelty of this disease, perhaps, is how ruthlessly it cleaves the soon-to-be bereaved from those they love so dearly.

Sally falls into bed with a child's abandon. From the arc of her spine to the soles of her feet, her entire body aches with exhaustion. She could happily lie under this duvet for weeks, yet sleep, when it comes, is fitful. A pale face flits in and out of her consciousness. The wide eyes. The straps of the mask on his cheeks. Her anxiety that the final experience of his life may end up being one of terror. She felt so proud of her team. Together, they have given a critically ill patient a chance at life. But doubt creeps in as she dozes. She tries to suppress what she knows: that the disease is so new and they understand so little.

Like Sally, Laura Wood is an intensive care nurse in Yorkshire. At twenty-four, she has been a nurse for a little over two years. Laura loves the ICU. Initially, upon qualifying, she found the relentless pressures of understaffing and lack of beds crushed her nursing ideals as she was forced to adapt to perpetual fire-fighting. ICU, on the other hand, with its rarefied ratios of one nurse to one or, at most, two patients, offered the chance to be the professional she had dreamed of being at nursing school. Focused. Absorbed. Meticulous and tireless. Never leaving things to chance, never slapdash. She has learned so much during her year on the unit, sometimes she still can't believe her luck to have arrived here.

Covid, however, is uncharted territory. Her ICU has never known so many critically unwell patients arrive so quickly and in such astonishing numbers. The intubations are as tense as any she has known. Laura hopes and prays she will only ever know this disease professionally, and not through personal experience.

Two hundred miles south of his daughter, Ken Wood, who lives with his wife in a small town in Oxfordshire, is unusually well primed against infection. Although he's just over sixty and fit – he likes his 10-kilometre runs to take less than an hour – the new virus from China is at the forefront of his mind. As the director of crisis management for an international food packaging company, Ken's work takes him all over the world. Since January, his company has been tracking the pandemic. As early as February, on business in Brazil, Ken set an example to other staff by wearing a face mask and practising social distancing.

Weeks before Britain is placed under lockdown, Ken takes the precaution of buying masks for his family and pays meticulous attention to handwashing. But then, on 17 March at eleven o'clock precisely, Ken hears the ring of the front doorbell. Once a week, at exactly this time, a dear friend has been visiting for years. In his eagerness to greet him – and with an uncharacteristic lapse of concentration – Ken instinctively leans forward, palm outstretched. As they shake hands, he kicks himself for ignoring his rules of physical distancing and makes a mental note to wash his hands immediately. But the conversation, as so often with old friends, is instantly beguiling. Distracted and buoyant, Ken sits down to chat, his usual fastidiousness forgotten. He would have thought nothing more of it except that, two days later, his friend telephones. 'I thought I should let you know, Ken. I'm feeling rotten and I have a fever. Just in case you start to feel ill too. It's probably nothing but – you know.'

The day before Ken makes accidental physical contact with his friend – Monday, 16 March – the Prime Minister finally announces a change of tack. Ostensibly, the reason for the abrupt change of policy is the publication of new modelling from experts at Imperial College London. Their data show that if measures are maintained in their current form, 250,000 Britons are likely to die from coronavirus. Alarmingly, Imperial predicts that intensive care units will be overwhelmed by severely ill patients eight times over.

In fact, the data on estimated fatalities were presented to the government the preceding week. I can't help but wonder whether it is the weekend's bad publicity around herd immunity that has crystallised Boris Johnson's thinking. Not that I care. Like every doctor I know, I am desperate for one thing only: definitive action. In London by now, some hospitals are already at breaking point. I feel almost deranged with impatience. I can think of nothing else. For the love of God, will you please – *please* – just shut the country down?

In the first of what will now become daily televised press conferences, Johnson advises the British population to stay at home if we can: 'Now is the time for everyone to stop non-essential contact with others and to stop all unnecessary travel. We need people to start working from home where they possibly can. And you should avoid pubs, clubs, theatres and other such social venues.'

In a second major escalation of existing policy, he announces that entire households must now self-isolate for fourteen days at home, should any member of the household develop symptoms of coronavirus. That means not leaving the house for any reason at all, even buying food or essentials. Vulnerable individuals, such as the over-seventies, are also told they need to 'shield' themselves from the virus in complete isolation at home for a twelve-week period.

According to the head of the Imperial modelling team, Professor Neil Ferguson, these new interventions – comprising a more aggressive 'suppression' strategy – should drive down the estimated death toll to 20,000 or fewer. On camera, Johnson appears distinctly uneasy about their 'draconian' (as he describes it) nature, commenting: 'Many people, including millions of active people over seventy, may feel, listening to what I've just said, that there is something excessive about these measures. But I have to say I believe they are overwhelmingly worth it, to slow the spread of the disease, reduce the peak, to save lives, minimise suffering and to give our NHS the chance to cope.'

The remark betrays the breadth of the disconnect between the government and frontline medics. That evening, my husband finds me at the kitchen table with my head in my hands. To me, what leaps out are the lacunae and lack of clarity. The messaging is mixed, its implications confusing. We have been advised not to visit pubs and restaurants, yet none of them have been ordered to close. Shops, gyms, hairdressers and schools all remain open. No travel restrictions have been enforced. Every restriction is optional, every suggestion voluntary. The advice is not remotely a lockdown. There is no insistence, no imposition and – crucially – no sanctions, even as some of London's intensive care units are buckling. As if to underline the inconsistency of the Prime Minister's position, his father promptly announces he will be ignoring him. 'Of course I'll go to the pub if I need to go to a pub,' Stanley Johnson declares on live breakfast television.

Two days later, the government at last announces that the country's schools will close at the end of the week for all but the children of key workers. My relief, however, is short-lived. At around the same time, the bleak news breaks in the *Health Service Journal* that Northwick Park Hospital in Harrow has been forced to declare a critical incident after running out of ICU beds. Soaring numbers of Covid patients have overwhelmed the hospital, which has been forced to transfer critically ill patients to neighbouring hospitals. This is precisely the chaos we were aghast to witness unfolding in Lombardy – only now it has arrived on our doorstep. Speaking of the Northwick Park critical incident, a senior manager at another London trust tells the journal it raises serious concerns about the ability of the capital's hospitals to deal with the surge in patients. The manager's assessment is uncompromising: 'Given we're in the low foothills of this virus, this is fucking petrifying.'

The same day, unpublished NHS figures obtained by the *Guardian* newspaper show that the number of people confirmed or suspected to have Covid being treated in ICUs in south London has risen from only 7 on 6 March to 93 on 17 March. A thirteen-fold increase in eleven days – and still the country isn't locked down. I receive a message from Arjun, my London colleague in infectious diseases, that makes me want to roar with rage: 'Everything exploding now. Patients coming out of our ears. It's basically Lombardy, it's insane.'

I lie awake every night now, body coiled, mind ticking. My PPE fitting at my local hospital took place on the same day I received a message from another colleague in London: 'We now have a doctor with Covid intubated in our ICU.' The words stung. The NHS is more than the sum of its parts. I am animated at work, for example, by deep loyalty to its founding principles, by my pride in inhabiting a society which sees that caring collectively for the health of those in need, regardless of their status, power or ability to pay, is a measure of basic human decency. I feel a kindred closeness to my fellow frontline staff, all the way from Edinburgh to Exeter. I know we are likely to share the same ideals, the same frustrations, the same gaps in the rotas, the same peeling ceilings, the same risk of burnout, the same threadbare wards, the same prehistoric IT and – above all – the same determination, when confronted with challenges, to rise to meet them for the sake of our patients. The thought of another member of my sprawling, teeming NHS family now lying intubated in an ICU fills me with anguish. Doctors and nurses sign up to save other people's lives, not to endanger their own.

But there is, I remind myself, something to cling on to. There is reason to hope. For all the dithering over when to commit to lockdown, in wards and clinics and general practices and operating theatres up and down the length of Britain a kind of grassroots revolution is underway. Decisions are being made, at breakneck speed, from the ground up. The 'lumbering', 'monolithic', 'bureaucratic' NHS that some armchair critics are only too eager to criticise is transforming itself with striking agility.

Oxford University Hospitals NHS Foundation Trust, like England's other 216 acute hospital, ambulance, community and mental health trusts, is throwing everything it has at creating ICU capacity. Collectively, the NHS's acute trusts employ 800,000 staff and treat over a million patients every thirty-six hours. Large hospital trusts can have annual budgets of over £1.5 billion and employ up to 20,000 staff. Running them requires a fiendishly complex support infrastructure equivalent in size to that of a small town, including oxygen, power, catering, laundry, patient transport and cleaning. Covid demands the complete transformation of every single part – not in months, nor weeks, nor even in days, but now, right now, as the tidal wave bears down.

Even the best-funded health service in the world could never accommodate a pandemic overnight. Yet the NHS is particularly wrong-footed, having been hollowed out by a decade of austerity budgets. In Oxford, for example, the A&E department quickly realises it needs some kind of outdoor pod where people with potential coronavirus who have travelled from high-risk countries can wait until a doctor emerges, in top-to-toe PPE, to escort them inside to an isolation room. But there are no pods and no money to buy them – and besides, the need is urgent. Which is how, at one stage, the department searches for and identifies for their purposes a sufficiently large garden shed from a major DIY chain. At the eleventh hour, the delivery of said B&Q shed to the hospital forecourt is averted when someone procures through dark magic an emergency Portakabin.

I receive a frantic message from a friend, Sarah, who works in another part of the country as a consultant psychiatrist. 'Are you OK in the midst of Armageddon, Rach? We've just been told our psych ward is going to be used for end-of-life Covid patients and we've no idea what to do. Panicking. Help.' Inpatient psychiatric units are not, to say the least, experienced in the management of acutely unwell patients dying from a lethal infectious disease. My offer to help leads me, forty-eight hours later, to be sitting at my kitchen table having an emergency Zoom meeting with several dozen psychiatrists from various parts of the country. Sarah's anxieties were clearly shared. At one point, I discover that none of these doctors have any idea how to safely put on or take off their PPE. No one has trained them. So I improvise, grabbing a pair of bright yellow Marigolds from the kitchen sink to give a live demonstration of the safest technique for glove removal. This is absolute madness, I tell myself.

Everything is scrambled, a race against the clock. Such is

the fear that the NHS will run out of ventilators, the Prime Minister invokes the spirit of Dunkirk in a direct appeal to the nation's engineers to redesign new ventilators from scratch. Shrewdly, Oxford's hospitals decide not to hold out for as yet back-of-the-envelope prototypes, instead wheeling and dealing with impressive zeal to access every additional tried-and-tested model they can. One of the trust's senior doctors becomes the de facto chief of pandemic procurement, negotiating furiously with local businesses, scientists, charities and transport chains to source masks, visors, gowns and ventilators. Rarely is this process straightforward and occasionally it descends into bio-medical farce.

On one occasion, a colleague tells him he's just had an offer from Oxford University: 'They're keen to do anything they can to help us. No barriers, no admin, they'll give us whatever they have that could be useful. They've been absolutely brilliant.'

The procurement chief follows up the lead and ends up speaking to a local university professor who thinks he may have just what the hospital needs.

'It's ventilators we're desperate for,' says the doctor. 'Ideally proper ICU ventilators but even anaesthetic machines are useful. We need every single one we can get.'

'Let me come back to you ASAP,' replies the academic, genuinely delighted that the university has a chance to play its part. 'I know exactly who to contact.'

The return phone call does not quite go to plan. The local university physiology department sometimes conducts experiments on animals. 'Good news!' the professor cries. 'We've got one! We can give you one ventilator. It's designed for . . . a macaque monkey.'

Macaques, the second most widespread primate on Earth, are typically around 10 kilograms in weight, the average size of a human toddler. The university's offer, while kind, is ill-suited to an adult intensive care unit. The procurement chief comments to me later: 'You know you are desperate when you are actually looking at a second-hand monkey ventilator and thinking, Is there any way we can use this?'

ICU is a precious, costly and scarce resource, reserved for the tiny number of critically ill patients at any one moment in a population. The UK's 4000 critical care beds mean that, when compared to other European countries, we are ranked only twenty-fourth out of thirty-one. We have four times fewer ICU beds per head of population than Germany, and ten times fewer than the US.

Every hospital in the UK is therefore tearing up rules and demolishing conventions to double or even treble its ICU capacity. All hands on deck, a national emergency. In my trust, the message is blunt: based on the information coming out of Italy, we need to prepare for twenty ICU admissions a day, four times what is normal. 'How the fuck are we going to do that?' says one senior manager. Another looks up, entirely calm. 'We have a major incident policy. We follow it. We cancel all elective surgery. We flow everything through ED. We use theatres, recovery rooms, we pull the staff from everywhere we can.'

Too many times in recent years – after the Grenfell fire, the Manchester Arena bombing, and London's Westminster Bridge and Borough Market terror attacks – the country has exhaled with pride and gratitude at the emergency responses of our NHS, police and fire services. These seemingly instantaneous acts of coordinated teamwork take months of rehearsal and planning. NHS trauma centres, for example, periodically enact full-scale major incidents, right down to teams of staff awash with fake blood, simulating with gusto the maimed and mangled. If the basics are wrong in a major incident – a chaotic triage of casualties, for example – people may die unnecessarily, their injuries fatally exacerbated by something as mundane as disorganisation.

I think back to the Westminster Bridge attack when, shortly after 2.30 p.m. on 22 March 2017, a car turned on to the bridge and began to accelerate in the direction of the Houses of Parliament. On the pavements, beneath unseasonably warm blue skies, briefcases jostled with selfie sticks and mobiles as locals rushed to be somewhere as quickly as possible, while tourists dawdled for photos, striking poses in the shadow of Big Ben.

The car, steered by a fifty-two-year-old Briton named Khalid Masood, mounted the pavement and began careering, deliberately, into the pedestrians. He was aiming for maximum carnage and left bodies strewn in his wake. One woman died immediately after being hit and thrown under the wheels of a bus, another as she walked past a stand selling postcards. Masood now crashed his vehicle into the perimeter of the Palace of Westminster, abandoning the car, pulling a seven-inch knife from his jacket, and running towards an unarmed policeman, PC Keith Palmer, on duty at the entrance. He fatally stabbed Palmer before being killed himself by a bullet fired by another, armed, policeman. The entire attack, from start to finish, lasted eighty-two seconds.

At the moment when Masood started mowing down

Londoners, the nursing director of one of London's three major trauma centres, St Mary's Hospital, was inside the chief executive's office, chairing a tense meeting about understaffing. Like most NHS hospitals in the capital, the staff vacancy rate was running between 12 and 14 per cent, and senior colleagues were discussing how they could possibly fill the 699 empty posts Mary's faced at the time.

Someone's phone rang. Then someone else's. Faces stiffened. By complete chance, a BBC film crew was inside the meeting, cameras rolling, as the news was relayed from the London Ambulance Service that a major incident had occurred. While quietly documenting staffing issues for the BBC2 series *Hospital*, the television crew thus found themselves capturing the tension and drama of a major NHS trauma centre's unfolding response to a terrorist attack.

At this point, though paramedics were being frantically mobilised, no one officially dispatched by the NHS had reached the scene of the attack. But a friend of mine, an off-duty NHS doctor called Jeeves Wijesuriya, happened to be inside a building located just around the corner from Parliament. As hundreds of people stampeded in panic away from Westminster Bridge, a woman burst into the building. Jeeves, a junior doctor in training to become a general practitioner, heard her scream, 'Someone's been shot! There's a shooting! I need to hide. Can I hide in the back of the building?' Jeeves looked out of the door to see a wall of people running. Instinctively, knowing that his training could save lives, Jeeves rushed into the mêlée to help. Pushing through the crowds towards a policeman, he said, 'I'm a doctor. Is everyone OK? Can I help?' The policeman immediately spoke into his radio and two undercover officers appeared out of the chaos, saying, 'Right, are you the doctor? We need you to come with us now.'

While officers herded the public away, Jeeves and the two plain-clothed agents sprinted towards the Palace of Westminster, the policemen's badges held high as they shouted, 'He's the doctor, the doctor! Let us through.'

On reaching the front entrance to Parliament, one of the officers pointed to a car and said to Jeeves, 'You need to know we're checking the area for additional devices and this is probably a terror attack.' Later, Jeeves would tell me about his response: 'You just have to put that out of your mind. So, I binned that information and went on. You just adopt your role. Literally, all I was thinking at this point was, Where is my patient? I need to treat my patient.'

Jeeves now came face to face with the aftermath of terror. Khalid Masood and Keith Palmer were both lying motionless on the ground before him. 'I saw two bodies, a knife on the ground, people doing chest compressions,' he told me. 'There were no ambulances, no paramedics, no equipment, nothing. I walked straight over thinking, Right, what's going on? Give me the key information about what's happened here. Don't tell me about second shooters, just tell me what I need to know. What's happened? One of the police officers said to me, "This is the police officer. He's been stabbed twice. And over there is the guy who did it. He's been shot by us. They're both in bad shape."'

Jeeves immediately started to assess the patients. It was as though he, the police officers and Tobias Ellwood, the Member of Parliament and former soldier who also gave Keith Palmer chest compressions, were an impromptu NHS crash team. 'I began by assessing the officer, checking for a pulse, assessing the quality of the compressions. I checked for a cardiac output but there was no pulse. I made sure people swapped in and out of compressions before they got tired. And I asked for more equipment – anything they had, cannulas, lines, fluids – but someone said, "Here, this is all we've got," and handed me a pair of blue plastic gloves. Seriously. Having none of the stuff we needed made me feel so bad, so powerless, but I figured, well, I'm trained. I'm more comfortable in this situation than these other guys are, so I just need to keep calm and do the basics, getting good oxygen, making sure we did the best life support possible, and trying to find a shockable rhythm.'

For six long minutes, Jeeves was the only NHS professional at the scene of the attack. 'They felt like five years,' he told me. When he asked if ambulances were on their way, the police informed him there were still fears of a bomb. 'Again, I just binned the implications of that.' There was, he said, simply no option of being frightened. 'There was just no time for that. And anyway, I couldn't be scared, I was in charge. We needed a doctor in charge, so I just had to be the doctor. Nobody realised I was just this random junior doctor – a GP trainee who happened to be nearby and offered to help.'

As soon as the paramedics arrived, Jeeves was so relieved to see another health professional that the first thing he blurted out was: 'Do you have equipment? We need equipment. Get your gear out!' The fact was, he admitted to me later, you could never feel more naked as a doctor than he did in those first six minutes, with nothing, no equipment, and two critically injured patients.

While the air ambulance team attended to Keith Palmer, Khalid Masood was whisked into an ambulance and blue-lighted straight to St Mary's Hospital. As the team, including Jeeves, ran with Masood on a stretcher into A&E, the BBC film crew was there, recording everything as it happened. Jeeves is seen at the front of the blood-soaked trolley, still giving chest compressions. The trauma team stands assembled, calmly awaiting the first casualty. Jeeves' handover to the lead consultant was not broadcast. 'We've done fifty-seven minutes of CPR, and in my view this man is dead,' Jeeves told him. Time of death was called almost immediately by the Mary's team, who then – entirely appropriately – simply turned their attention to receiving the next casualty.

Years of meticulous planning for major trauma at Mary's were coming into their own. 'When a major incident happens, within twelve minutes the entire hospital has kicked into a completely different way of working,' said Dr Alison Sanders, clinical director at Imperial College Healthcare NHS Trust, to the BBC cameras. 'We have to do something entirely different, with zero notice, and you see everybody just switch into it.'

Among those stepping up instantly to receive the casualties was one of Mary's most experienced and trusted trauma anaesthetists, Helgi Johannsson. He recounted to me afterwards the commonplace nature of catastrophe to a trauma team. 'We were calm that day because, quite simply, it's what we do every day. I stopped being scared of terrorist activity a long, long time ago. There was no reason to panic or shout and scream because we deal with so many sad stories and horrific injuries. This wasn't any different. You see personal tragedies all the time in this job – people who just happen to be in the wrong place, at the wrong time – and you learn how arbitrary and precarious life is.'

Unlike the rest of us, who tend to live our lives in denial of calamitous bolts from the blue, a major trauma centre predicts and prepares for the unthinkable – and it showed. The BBC cameras captured the slick composure of Mary's staff clearing every patient they could from the hospital to make space for the influx of victims. Despite the hospital's usual overcrowding and understaffing, nothing would slow the treatment of the incoming victims.

Helgi chose to describe it to me in earthier terms: 'A major incident instantly turns the hospital from a clusterfuck upon clusterfuck of capacity problems into an amazing, efficient, massive machine. We have a brilliant major incident plan. We cleared all our elective surgery immediately. A fleet of ambulances rushed to the hospital to take away everyone who was well enough to be treated in a standard hospital rather than a major trauma centre. Our ITU colleagues from Charing Cross and Hammersmith hospitals came in more ambulances to take away anyone in our ITU who was well enough to be transferred. That freed up our ITU capacity as well. In a matter of minutes, so quickly, we had capacity to take thirty, forty, fifty patients.'

In a major trauma, it is effective logistics, more than anything else, that saves lives. Training, planning and relentless practice – systems that work under fire. But even trauma physicians are human. 'Every once in a while that night, I'd have to go and stand in a corner, pause briefly and take a long deep breath,' Helgi told me. There was one point, while resuscitating an American tourist, Melissa Cochran – in London with her husband, Kurt, to celebrate their twenty-fifth wedding anniversary – when Helgi felt flooded with anger. Unbeknown to his critically injured wife, Kurt had been killed on the bridge. A postcard of the Queen among Melissa's belongings, purchased that day as a small souvenir, caught her doctor's eye.

'It hit me then,' Helgi told me. 'This was the moment a theoretical incoming "casualty" became a person, a human being who had been admiring Big Ben, walking along holding hands with a now-dead husband. When I saw the postcard of the Queen, it seemed to sum it all up for me. This was a deliberate attack on the nation, the head of the nation, and a disrespect to everyone in the nation. A nasty, calculated, vindictive thing to do to all of us. And we couldn't let it divide us. We couldn't allow to happen what the attacker wanted to happen. We couldn't allow London to empty, people to stay at home under curfew. I felt all of that right then.'

The unassuming bravery displayed by Jeeves and Helgi that day was by no means unique. As their phones lit up with live news of the terror attack, staff streamed out from another hospital, St Thomas's, positioned directly opposite the Houses of Parliament. Tommy's doctors and nurses sprinted across Westminster Bridge to help the casualties, joining the hundreds of police officers who were already there, endangering their lives in turn.

The NHS has no monopoly on selflessness, as the Westminster attack admirably demonstrates. *Every* first responder – police, paramedic, doctor, firefighter – took profound risks that day in order to save others. So too did many ordinary citizens, individuals with neither training nor experience, only their altruistic drive. Yet, it is hard to imagine another British institution more densely packed with the best of human nature – bravery, tolerance, cooperation, kindness – than the

NHS in London that day. For Helgi, the profound sense of purpose the attack provided transcended the anger it simultaneously stirred. 'In a bizarre way, I absolutely loved working that night. Obviously, it was awful in one sense, but I knew we were providing really excellent clinical care to those patients. The team atmosphere was incredible. Our morale as a hospital was as high as it has ever been in the whole history of Mary's. We were doing something important, that mattered, and we were doing it really well. And, yes, we were angry at the perpetrator, but we were also overwhelmingly proud of our response as a hospital.'

Health administrators rarely earn public plaudits. Indeed, the NHS is sometimes depicted in the British press as an institution managed by bungling incompetents who squander resources like confetti. Yet on this day, hidden far away from the trauma team heroics, scores of NHS officials in the capital's major incident control room worked around the clock – as they had trained to do for years – to ensure that all of London's NHS organisations had enough resources to deal with the attack, and that the most seriously injured went to the hospitals best equipped to help them. One of them told the *Guardian* newspaper: 'This was a serious incident and it's incredibly sad what's happened. But this sort of incident is what the NHS is ready for, especially in London. It's one of the best places in the world for providing a quick, organised emergency response to a terrorist incident. People talk all the time about the NHS being under pressure, which it is. But when this sort of thing happens, you can't beat the NHS.'

Much later, Jeeves confronted the idea that he could have been killed at the scene of the attack. 'I did think later, what if I'd died?' he told me, but only because I asked. 'If I had died there, I would have died doing what I'm trained to do. I would have gone out doing something decent for people who were hurt, and my parents probably would have come to terms eventually with it being a pretty decent thing for their son to have done.'

The pandemic is the first *nationwide* major incident in NHS history. But instead of lasting eighty-two seconds, this is an incident with no end in sight. Local teams across the country are working with urgency and passion to do whatever is needed to save as many lives as they can. Hospitals are reinventing themselves with astonishing alacrity. All non-urgent surgery is suspended, just as it would be in a local major incident. Operating theatres, recovery areas, normal wards and even conference rooms are transformed into ersatz ICUs. Psychiatrists, surgeons, rheumatologists and medical students are pulled from their day jobs to help staff them day and night, often with little more than a day's emergency training. Logistics become matters of life and death. Every hospital has to be sure it will not run out of oxygen – as has happened, unimaginably, in Lombardy. A London conference hall mutates in nine days into the first of a series of NHS Nightingale hospitals, this one alone capable of receiving 4000 additional patients in need of intensive care.

The first patients with coronavirus arrived in Oxford's John Radcliffe Hospital in February. They presented to the ED with severe pneumonias only subsequently diagnosed as Covid. Three weeks later, by the first week of March, the entire first floor of the hospital had been dissected into red and blue zones. One

Monday morning, the trust's divisional director responsible for ED, intensive care, acute medicine and anaesthetics gathered his team for an emergency presentation. A particular slide in the PowerPoint leapt out, an architect's drawing of the reconstructed first floor, with a thick line neatly segregating red from blue.

'When I saw that, I felt so relieved,' one of the ED consultants, David Pritchard, tells me. 'We've known winters when we don't just run out of beds, we run out of corridor space. I couldn't see how we'd have the space for the numbers we were expecting. But the plan was radical, brilliantly so. Our capacity was being transformed.'

Red tape has gone down – literally – all over the first floor. But this tape, instead of stultifying and hampering, cleanly carves so-called 'Respiratory' from 'Non-Respiratory' ED – our euphemisms of choice for Covid and non-Covid. New doors, partitions and screens go up overnight. 'You know,' says David drily, 'the kind of thing that in the NHS normally takes twenty-six committees and two years to achieve.' He goes on: 'It is mind-blowing, exhilarating, the empowerment of being able to do everything necessary to make it work – with money, for once, no object – and everyone working together to do what is right.'

Staff are simultaneously resolute and fearful. 'I really don't have any desire to be a hero,' David tells me. 'I'm not exactly scared of dying, but I can't bear the thought of leaving my children. I am married to another doctor. We both know there is a chance we are going to turn our kids into orphans.'

In the ICU, staff have been told to prepare for a total number of intubated Covid patients at any one time that might reach 150. But this is in a hospital whose adult ICU normally contains only sixteen beds. In one meeting of senior clinicians, one asks, 'Well, what are we going to do?'

The stark truth is that squeezing extra beds into the adult ICU will never match demand. The paediatric ICU, the cardio-thoracic critical care unit and every theatre recovery space may need to be taken over as well. All eyes turn to the clinical lead for intensive care, whose reply is as frank as it is blunt: 'We have no other option. We'll just have to do our best.'

Everyone is trying to magic beds from thin air. Even my little hospice plays its part with aplomb. In less than a fortnight, a crack squad of builders transforms us from a ten-bedded traditional hospice into the twenty-six-bedded 'Katharine House Response Centre' – ready and waiting to care for infected and non-infected patients alike. We have become, in essence, a field hospice. Our casualties will be brought here from home, hospital, care homes – anywhere – and we will welcome them all.

I am aware it is our nurses and carers who will be most exposed to potential infection. For though the caring bit of healthcare is often seen through misty eyes – as hand holding, thoughtful gestures and going the extra mile – care is inescapably visceral. Kindness, undeniably, is the glue that ensures patients feel safe and hospitals humane. But care is tough too, sometimes brutally so. Care, on occasion, can be wiping blood and vomit from a patient as they squirm in fear. Care is scooping someone up from the floor of the bathroom where they lie coated in their own diarrhoea. Care is catheters, stoma bags, pus and urine. Care can stink and overpower. My colleagues' skill at providing this most intimate of services – with unfailing tenderness and patience – has never failed to astound me. But it also puts them at particular risk of infection.

With the numbers of dead doctors and nurses in Italy steadily rising, the potential dangers of caring for Covid patients are very far from theoretical. Indeed, when Charlie Bond, the hospice medical director, asks the nursing team how they might feel about looking after those known to be infected, they discuss those risks among themselves with furious intensity. I am there when the nurses and carers tell him their answer. Lisa, the most senior nurse on the ward that day, gives the team's considered opinion. 'We've talked about it and we don't care what we do, Charlie. We just want to stay together as a team. And we want to do whatever helps most.'

Charlie blinks for a moment and I have to look down so Lisa cannot catch my eye. When he responds, his voice is thick with emotion. 'Someone mentioned to me earlier that most of all you wanted to stay as a team. I was very moved. You've really shown amazing compassion and courage.'

Across the whole of the UK, the scale of change is unprecedented in the NHS's seventy-two-year history. In under a month, a total of 33,000 extra patient beds are created – the equivalent of building fifty-three new district general hospitals across the country. Dave Jones, an ICU consultant in Wales, posts a tweet that makes us grin in wry recognition: 'The NHS reminds me of a hippopotamus. It might sometimes appear slow, maybe a bit bloated and somewhat unresponsive. But my god, this last week or so has shown that like a hippo, it can move bloody fast and have some awesome power when it needs to.'

There will be, we shall learn in due course, a terrible cost to the NHS's single-minded focus, however necessary it may be. On 17 March, the same day that Northwick Park Hospital runs out of beds, government ministers publish new hospital discharge guidance that requires 15,000 hospital beds to be vacated by 27 March. At any one time, up to 30 per cent of NHS patients are medically fit to be discharged from hospital, yet unable to leave because it has not been possible to ensure appropriate social care is in place for them. Making their beds available is part of a 'national effort' that will 'help to save thousands of lives', says the document. The intention – both admirable and necessary – is to protect Covid patients from a scenario similar to the ongoing devastation in northern Italy, where hospitals are overwhelmed. But the government insists in formal Department of Health and Social Care guidance that there is no need to test hospital patients for Covid prior to discharge because even those who are infected 'can be safely cared for in a care home'. At the time, with the crisis in Northwick Park revealing how closely we are teetering towards the unthinkable prospect of having to ration care and deny patients ventilators, I do not think to question that phrase. It is an assertion, based less on evidence than on wishful thinking, that will come back to haunt every one of us.

Ken Wood, the father of ICU nurse Laura, had hoped that the call from his friend whose hand he'd accidentally shaken would end up amounting to nothing. That same day, Ken visits the gym as normal, taking to the treadmill for 10 brisk kilometres as usual. But the next day he wakes up feeling hot and shivery. The injustice of it smarts a little. He has been wearing a mask and washing his hands religiously since well before lockdown was even underway. He is a man who spent over £100 on state-of-the-art masks for his family.

Initially, he insists — to himself as much as to Helen, his wife — that his symptoms are nothing more than a cold. But he finds himself spending more and more time sprawled on the sofa, poleaxed by something that is clearly more virulent. When his temperature soars to 39.5°C, Helen calls the 111 NHS helpline and a GP writes a remote prescription for antibiotics and steroids. The pills do nothing at all. Ken languishes at home, coughing and sweating. Laura and Helen wonder how worried they should be.

By day six of Ken's symptoms, his family are deeply concerned. Laura video-calls her mother and sees Dad in the background, listlessly sprawled on the sofa. His jeans, Laura notices, with a nurse's attentiveness, are not even done up properly. This is not her father, whose standards are unsparing. His posture and his dishevelment are red flags. She discusses what she's observed with Helen, who is herself a retired nurse. 'Mum,' she says, 'what do you think? Do you think you should call 111 again? He just doesn't look well. Please will you let me know what his pulse and his temperature are as you check them?'

A few days later, Ken's temperature soars again. At times, he barely seems to make sense when he speaks. His words are less slurred than incoherent. It is a Saturday and Laura asks work for permission to take Sunday off in order to be there for her father. She will still be a whole 200 miles away but at least, by phone, she can support her mother. Her ICU is understanding and permits the urgent leave with one proviso: if they become overwhelmed — the Covid patients are arriving thick and fast now — she may have to return for her Sunday day shift.

That Sunday, Ken seems to rally a little. He even manages to converse intelligibly in the morning with Laura. She tells herself he has turned a corner. You want to convince yourself your loved ones are safe. *It cannot be Dad. Not someone so healthy.* This isn't something that could happen to her family.

Laura is summoned with apologies to work. The ICU is reeling from the number of new Covid admissions overnight and they cannot do without her. By the time she returns from the hospital that evening, her mother is cautiously optimistic. 'I'm off to bed,' Laura tells her. 'Please will you call me if Dad deteriorates?'

It is only long after Laura falls asleep that Ken's temperature begins to rise again. At midnight, it approaches 40°C. His chest hurts every time he tries to leave the sofa. His wife calls 111 who this time take no chances. An ambulance is dispatched, sirens blaring. Ken is well aware of how vulnerable people can be to injury and disease, yet still cannot quite believe he is seriously unwell. He greets the paramedics, obscured behind their masks, with a smile. He manages to walk unaided, defiant, to the ambulance. He turns and peers back through the darkness to Helen, who stands wanly in a pool of yellow light on the doorstep. 'I'll see you later,' he assures her blithely. He isn't anxious. He imagines this is a sensible precaution, and he'll be home in a day or so.

In the morning, Laura wakes up to six missed calls on her mobile, all of them from her mother. Her adrenalin surges so abruptly, so viciously, her trembling fingers can hardly press the buttons.

'Mum? Mum? What's happened? Is Dad OK?'

Her mother's voice sounds so small on the end of the phone. Almost a whisper, infused with apology. 'Your dad's in intensive care, Laura. They moved him there at four o'clock this morning. His lungs weren't working. They needed to keep a close eye on him. They're doing all they can. I've asked them to call you to tell you how he is. I know you understand it all better than I do.'

Laura can scarcely comprehend that someone as relatively young and fit as her father could require intensive care. There is no one like him in her own ICU. This is not who coronavirus claims. She screws her eyes tightly shut, as if to blot out the news, and fights to keep her voice calm. 'I'll pack now, Mum,' she says. 'I'll drive down straight away.' She knows only too well what Covid can do to a body. To think of her father so reduced, so overthrown and vulnerable, is almost too painful to bear.

It is like this now, up and down the country. People are being swept from their homes in the darkness, rushed by paramedics to the nearest hospital. Their loved ones don't know it – the realisation is yet to dawn – but this may be the last time they will ever set eyes on them. You wave your goodbyes, you declare your love on the doorstep, you close the front door as the sirens start shrieking, and you wait and wait for news from inside the hospital.

6

The Thin Red Line

*In the face of fear, we are all starlings, a group, a flock, made
of a million souls seeking safety.*

HELEN MACDONALD, *Vesper Flights*

Ken is being raced through the night along a dual carriageway,
his eyes looking up at the roof of the ambulance. The gleaming,
the starkness, the thin fluorescent lights above, he studies it all
with quiet approval. He notes the glass-doored, head-height
cupboards packed with bottles, boxes, packets and bags, all
these medical essentials arranged as neatly as eggs in a nest.
There is bleeping and flashing, digital numbers on the run.
Everything speaks of deftness and precision. He could drift, he
could cast off, he is sure he's in safe hands.

The paramedic in the back knows to keep her patient talking. As she fits the oxygen mask over Ken's face, she keeps
on chatting, reassuring him. The severity of Ken's hypoxia
is reflected not one jot in his calmness and ease. By now, the
paramedic has seen a few like him already. Oxygen saturations

at 60 per cent on room air. Chatting when they should be thrashing for air. Behind her mask and gown, the paramedic's expression can't be read. Yet as she concentrates on conveying quiet authority, inside she is thinking for the hundredth time, What exactly is this thing we are dealing with?

Ken peers up at new faces, new streaks of fluorescence. More masks, more visors that gleam in the bleached light. His trolley weaves at speed along an unseen scarlet line and, when he enters the Respiratory ED, he passes rows of chairs on which more patients sit in masks. These are the less critical new arrivals with suspected Covid, the ones who can wait their turn. Eyes pivot like magnets on to his face, then whip away as though one glance could be fatal. Ken feels giddy and dazed, a specimen in transit. He secretly suspects he will be home in the morning, though his composure briefly wavers as he thinks of his wife alone. People approach. Questions are asked. He smiles and answers each one as best he can. He wants them to know he appreciates everyone. And he does. They are brilliant, his shrouded saviours.

A doctor appears, or maybe a nurse. She seems young and friendly, though with her visor and mask it is hard to tell. Warm anyway, kind in her manner. 'We're going to give you an injection,' she tells him. He surrenders his body with neither premonition nor fear. That offensive phrase, happy hypoxia. But he *is* confident. Like Laura, his daughter, they will know exactly what to do. The strip lights flicker, the clangs and bleeps start to fade. He remembers nothing more, he is gone.

The morning after Ken arrives in the ED, the emergency medicine consultant David Pritchard is showing me round. The department is unrecognisable from my time here as a junior doctor. First, we walk through the non-Covid side – 'Majors' as it used to be known. Ordinarily the place would be a maelstrom of sepsis and strokes, overdoses and haemorrhages, fizzing and bristling with patients' desperation. But today the moaning, shouting, swearing and sobbing – the typical soundtrack of a city ED – are replaced by an uncanny quiet.

'Where is everyone?' I ask David.

'We're really concerned,' he answers. 'They're keeping away, we're just not seeing them.'

The country is finally, mercifully, locked down. Only key workers are permitted to travel. The rest of the population are allowed outside only to exercise and to buy essential items like food. Anyone caught breaking the rules is liable to a police fine. But something more insidious than the law is keeping people inside. Fear of infection, of death by suffocation, is pinning people behind closed doors, too frightened to risk venturing outside, even when they feel unwell.

Covid's reach, it is evident, extends far beyond its human hosts, endangering not only the infected but the uninfected too. The patients we would usually expect in their droves in the ED have vanished, electing not to come. I imagine the sudden onset of chest pain at home in someone who smokes and has been warned about cardiac risk factors. He knows exactly what this pressure beneath his sternum could signify. He might even consider reaching for his phone. But why call 999 and risk becoming part of a future daily death toll, announced by some sombre-faced minister on live national television? Why not tough it out at home – take some paracetamol if necessary – enduring a transient discomfort that will surely pass? The government's messaging is actively urging such stoicism. Stay at home, we've been told repeatedly. Protect the NHS.

We reach a set of double doors emblazoned with red and white warning signs: 'STOP. Respiratory ED. Do not enter without appropriate PPE.' Once through, the atmosphere pulses with energy and tension. Staff stride between beds with a grim sense of purpose, any softness concealed beneath the carapace of gloves and gowns. Perched on plastic chairs, patients shrink behind their masks like wilting bandits. Their eyes search the department for comfort, for confidence, as they angle their bodies away from each other, curling into themselves.

These are the healthiest ones, sufficiently stable to await a full assessment. In the beds beyond the chairs lie the more gravely unwell. Here, the patients' masks are hooked with tubes to the wall, delivering ever-increasing concentrations of oxygen while their vital signs flicker on digital screens, the galloping heart rates and deoxygenated blood speaking of what may be to come. Long before any coronavirus test is back, their chest X-rays often confirm their doctor's fears. The virus presents itself time and again in the same unmistakable monochrome form. In the place of two clean air-filled lungs – reassuringly black, twin voids of air on the screen – are blotches and smears of thick white infection. It looks like raggedy fungus, left and right of the heart.

We walk past a side room, its doors firmly closed, and through the small square windows I glimpse a flash of activity inside. A patient lies prone – on his belly, limbs splayed – as three figures, visors bowed, work around his bed. The curve of his back is naked and white, one hand hangs from the sheet like an empty glove. I cannot tell if he is dead, unconscious or simply exhausted. A pair of eyes behind a visor briefly catches mine, and then we are gone.

I am here after pleading with the hospice bosses to let me join the hospital team. I cannot bear any longer this feeling of impotence while the country careers into the crisis in which Italy is already so painfully immersed. The only way I know of managing my fears is through action, trying to help, focusing on one patient, and then another, and then the one after that. It has been agreed that I can split my role, partly working with Covid patients on the wards of the hospital, partly caring for our hospice inpatients, who may have cancer, Covid, heart failure, liver disease, a perforated bowel or any of the other myriad conditions that can cut a life short.

Today, in the emergency department, some new recruits have been assembled and I've been asked to assist with their hastily arranged induction. The twenty-five freshest members of the ED team are so young and inexperienced they have yet to qualify as doctors. In the scramble to build capacity for the expected surge in patients, Oxford's medical school has asked its students whether they would like to help. The response has been an overwhelming yes. I feel immeasurably proud of them, our volunteer student army. They could have steered clear of the potential risk and trauma. Nobody would have thought less of them at all. Yet here they are, ready to do whatever they can to help, at whatever cost to themselves.

One of the students, Emma Flint, a twenty-four-year-old in her final year, had just embarked on what must surely be one of the world's most short-lived elective placements abroad. As she flew through the night around the world to Perth, Australia imposed a fourteen-day quarantine on all new arrivals.

She landed in the airport to discover that, while she had been in mid-air, she had effectively been placed under compulsory quarantine, with fines of $50,000 for venturing outside, even to go and buy groceries. Emma's ten-week adventure learning antipodean paediatrics turned into three dismal days locked down inside an Airbnb, living off Pot Noodles and cereal bars purchased from the airport shop. 'I did glimpse one kangaroo from the Uber,' she told me, 'and that was it, I flew straight back home again.'

Emma and her twenty-four fellow students are now sitting at home, glued to their laptops, as I commence an online teaching session from within the ED about death and dying in pandemic times. For me, Zoom is still an exotic novelty. I can't believe how easily we are able to interact, nor how fresh-faced and vulnerable the students seem on my screen.

I try to convey what it looks and sounds like to be dying of Covid. How quickly and remorselessly a patient can be overwhelmed. Which drugs we use to help ease their fear and hunger for air. How hard it is to convey warmth and humanity when trussed up behind a visor and mask. The cost for patients and families of being kept apart. The cost for us, the clinicians, of having to enforce these estrangements. All the while I watch the students' faces as I try to steer a path between alarming them and supporting them. When I was twenty-four, I knew nothing. This feels like a crash course in mortal reckoning. We should not be sitting miles apart.

'Even at the best of times, palliative care can be tough,' I say. 'There are moments when you can feel overwhelmed with sadness. But now patients are alone when they long for their loved ones. Everyone they see looks like an alien in a mask.

Conversations that should happen face to face, in person, have to take place over the phone. You find yourself telling an eighty-year-old woman that her husband is dying, knowing she is sitting in her bungalow alone. All of this is wrong, it feels as wrong as it is possible to be in medicine. Sometimes I have to make myself as hard as nails to do it. But that's OK, and it's OK if you find yourself wanting to cry sometimes too. It's normal, natural. You may have gone through medical school being taught that displaying emotion is weakness. It isn't. It's human. If you find things tough, please talk to your team. This is going to be hard for everyone.'

I am trying to give the students permission to feel. Many will have yet to see a patient die, even as they plunge into pandemic medicine. They need to know that shock, distress, fear and trepidation are not dirty secrets but normal human responses. Behind the scenes, I know that the ED is pulling out the stops to build a field psychological support service for *all* its frontline staff. I find the prescience deeply impressive. Not so long ago, the emotional toll of medicine and nursing on practitioners was largely brushed under the carpet.

Emma finds herself posted on the front doors to the ED. In pairs, the students use a flowchart to direct patients and paramedics to the appropriate part of the department, trying to sift the infected from the benign. Anyone coughing or feverish or struggling to breathe is told to follow the red line on the floor that snakes into the hot zone, where everyone has Covid until proven otherwise. Only those with convincingly non-Covid reasons to be arriving at a hospital – the broken-boned, burned or inebriated, for example – are dispatched along the blue line to uncontaminated areas. Swiftly, this sieving and dispatching of patients becomes straightforward. Infinitely harder is the task of vetting the loved ones who accompany the patients here, deciding who is permitted to enter, and who to send away. Disaster gatekeeping – this unprecedented severing of distraught family members from each other – is not a skill they teach in any hospital.

'The rules are so strict,' Emma later tells me. 'Basically, you are only allowed a visitor if you are a woman in labour, a young child, someone who is dying or someone who needs extra support, like a patient with dementia. Everyone else has to turn around and go.'

The visitor restrictions are a particular cruelty of Covid. They have been imposed with the very best of intentions – to protect as many people as possible from preventable infection – but they are as brutal as they are necessary. Emma recalls meeting a young woman who arrived at the hospital in the act of having a miscarriage, doubled over on the forecourt as her partner endeavoured to keep her upright. Both their faces were white as bone. 'I had to explain to them both that he couldn't stay,' Emma says. 'I knew this woman was going to have to complete her miscarriage by herself, completely alone in the department, behind a mask, and it felt like the opposite of everything I'd been taught as a medical student and I hated it.'

Once, a man appeared at the front doors after being called by the hospital to say that his mother, rushed in by ambulance a few hours earlier, was now dying from coronavirus inside. His words tumbled out, a torrent of beseeching: 'I know it's probably not possible, I know it can't be done, but I have to get as close as I can to her, even if all that means is the car park. Could you just ask if I might be allowed to see her? Just for a moment. So I can tell her I love her? I just need her to hear that.'

Emma disappeared into the Respiratory ED, promising to do what she could. She re-emerged, forgetting that a smile can't be seen behind a mask, and beamed as she offered to take him to his mother's bed. He never stopped talking as she helped him into his PPE. 'Thank you so much, this is so typical of the NHS. You're just brilliant, legends, all of you. I can't tell you, it means the world to me that I can be here at the end for my mum.'

The red line took them both through the double doors, past the hissing and beeping, the monitors and pipes, the urgent conversations, the bobbing masks. There, behind a curtain, her hair white and wild, lay his mother in a dishevelled hospital gown. Emma found a chair and quietly set it down at the head of the bed. Just before she turned away, she saw two eyelids flicker open above the oxygen mask; two hands in blue gloves enclose a gnarled set of fingers, moisture glints on the face of a grieving son.

Months before she is even meant to qualify as a doctor, what Emma is giving of herself to these families is, I am certain, priceless.

A short walk down the corridor from where I have been teaching is the adult ICU. Ken lies here now, though he doesn't know it. The moment he arrived in the ED, it was instantly apparent his situation was critical. The proliferation of whiteness on his chest X-ray was caused not primarily by Covid itself but by his immune system being triggered into over-zealous action. The white blood cells and chemicals that sought to fight the infection had spiralled out of control into a 'cytokine storm', causing severe inflammation in his already battered lungs.

Inflamed lungs leak fluid and, in Ken's case, this had poured from his capillaries to flood the spaces that should tremble with air. The architecture of his lungs, once a gossamer web, was a sodden mass. Every inhalation took place against that weight. Ken unconsciously recruited new muscles to help pull air into his lungs. His neck muscles tensed, the tissue between his ribs quivered and retracted inwards, his abdomen surged and dropped. Yet still the oxygen in his blood continued to fall. His lips were stained blue now, his fingertips dark. Ken's body was at war with itself.

When I was taught about autoimmune diseases as a student, I listened in awe at the ease with which the human immune system can destroy the very thing it has evolved to save. Some of the most feared and remorseless of diseases – multiple sclerosis, ulcerative colitis, systemic lupus erythematosus – occur when the body turns upon itself, destroying human cells it mistakes as foreign invaders. Something equally formidable seems to happen with Covid. At first, your immune system is your best chance of recovery, its cells marshalled to attack and wipe out every viral particle. For most people infected with Covid, that is the end of the matter. They rapidly recover from a mild illness, sometimes so inconsequential as to entirely pass them by. But in a small minority of patients, the immune system seems to become supercharged, causing severe inflammation in the lungs, heart, brain or kidneys – or every one of the main organs, a physiological catastrophe. Not only that, as doctors are rapidly learning, the virus disrupts the delicate balance of clotting agents in the blood, increasing its viscosity. Patients are put at risk of life-threatening blood clots. Covid, in short, is no mere flu or pneumonia. It can escalate into devastating multi-system organ failure to which even the youngest and most robust of patients may fatally succumb. All of this knowledge is being acquired on the run, in real time, as patients lurch from physiological crisis to crisis. Our ignorance – and impotence – can feel unbearable.

The ICU offers a last-ditch attempt at surviving Covid, essentially by using machines to perform the work of the vital organs that have failed. There is no more high-tech environment in medicine, yet intensive care is less a cure than a means of buying time, of temporarily replacing the functions of failing organs until, we hope, they manage to recover. Life support is precisely this – a mechanical strategy for providing oxygen and fluids and clearing waste as a body queasily lurches between life and death, held there only thanks to precision engineering. Highly trained specialist nurses monitor the patient's entire body around the clock. An electrocardiogram continuously tracks the heart while an arterial line assesses blood pressure, oxygen and carbon dioxide levels, and the finest details of blood chemistry. The slightest deterioration in a patient's physiology is picked up and acted upon instantly.

When Ken first arrived here, the ICU team hoped to avoid having to sedate and intubate him by using a continuous positive airway pressure (CPAP) device that boosts the pressure of the air inside the lungs to help keep them inflated. But even on CPAP, by the time dawn broke he was dangerously weak. The team was left with no choice. A doctor calmly assembled the kit she would need. The laryngoscope to visualise Ken's larynx, the drugs with which to sedate and immobilise him, the endotracheal tube she would thread down his airway. She moved to the head of the trolley upon which he lay and, with one syringe, induced a medical coma. With the next, she paralysed all the muscles of his body. He lay inert, a minute or two from death. Slickly, she inserted her airway. A ventilator now performed his work of breathing, inflating by force his water-clogged lungs and giving the muscles of his chest much-needed respite. As to whether he was dying, surviving or somewhere in between, no one in the room could say.

I unlock the front door and reach for the hand sanitiser. Before I have even rushed upstairs to the shower – this is Mum's new routine, every night she's home from work now – Dave appears in the hallway, looking stern. 'We need to talk,' he says.

My mind leaps compulsively to death and disaster. They have been there, after all, throughout my day on the wards. Dave's parents, my mum? Has someone succumbed and been rushed into hospital? 'No, no,' says Dave. 'It's Abbey. We just need to talk.'

As quickly as possible, I try to scrub every speck of infection from my skin beneath the shower. The water cannot be too hot nor too forceful. I know that on one level I am trying to erase what I have seen and heard and sought to palliate today – yet understand that these experiences, whether I like it or not, are indelible. Still damp, hair dripping, I find Dave and he explains what has happened.

'Abbey started to cry, Rach,' he tells me. 'She doesn't want you to do anything at work that could end up killing you.'

My head slumps into my palms. Finn was two years old when I became a doctor. Abbey was born during my second year of practice. In all that time, over and over, my children have suffered as the hospital has consumed too many hours, just too much of their mother. The anodyne phrase 'work-life balance' doesn't come close to capturing the forcefulness with which medicine clashes with parenthood. Who comes first, patient or child? How can you walk out on this young man who has just learned he has terminal cancer? How many more nights must your baby daughter fall asleep without seeing her mother?

At nine, Abbey likes nothing more than sloths, meerkats, candyfloss, toffee apples and being mercilessly sprayed with the garden hose. I oscillate between delighting in the grown-up girl she is evolving into – all gangling limbs and vehement opinions – and missing the tiny creature I once cuddled for hours. And now I have caused my daughter, this diminutive firecracker I love so fiercely, sufficient pain to reduce her to tears. She does not want her mother to die and she fears that – through my *choices*, my self-selected pyramid of people with importance – she may lose me to coronavirus. Who do I love the most? I can imagine her thinking. My son and my daughter – my actual children – or these men and women I have never even met before who happen, by chance, to be my patients?

'I'll talk to her,' I mutter to Dave, too ashamed to meet his eye. 'What I'm doing really isn't high risk. ICU is much more dangerous.'

Abbey and I sit on her bed behind closed doors. 'Hey,' I say gently, as she picks at the duvet. 'Dad said you got upset today?'

Her voice is harsh and hostile, completely out of character. 'Why do *you* have to be the one who sees all the coronavirus patients in the hospital? Why can't it be someone else who doesn't have children so if they die, it isn't as bad?'

I hesitate. How can I possibly tell her I have volunteered, that I *want* to be the one helping these patients? Yet equally, how can I lie to her? I take a deep breath and grope for the right words.

'Abbey,' I begin, 'I don't believe I am going to die. I think I may well have already had the virus.'

She cuts in before I can say more. 'Well, what if you're wrong? You don't know, do you?' Tears are forming in the corners of her eyes.

'You're right, I don't know. But I'm not working in the most dangerous part of the hospital. That's called intensive care, where the sickest patients are. I'm on the normal wards where it's not so risky.'

We debate back and forth as I try to articulate the nature of duty in terms a nine-year-old can understand, this irresistible tug to use my training to help in a crisis. 'Well, what about your duty to me? And to Finn?' she asks defiantly. The more I try to assure her I will be safe, the more stridently she insists I can't know that. And, of course, she's right. I can't. I cannot promise her the worst won't happen.

We reach an uneasy truce when I swear to be as careful as possible, avoiding high-risk areas if I can. As a mother, I'm not sure I have ever felt shabbier.

The same day I am teaching in A&E, the first UK doctor to die of coronavirus is named. Mr Amged El-Hawrani, a fifty-five-year-old ear, nose and throat consultant surgeon, died two days earlier in Leicester's Glenfield Hospital. A spokesperson for his family states: 'Amged was a loving and much-loved husband, son, father, brother, and friend. His greatest passions were his family and his profession, and he dedicated his life to both. He was the rock of our family, incredibly strong, compassionate, caring and giving. He always put everyone else before himself. We all turned to him when we needed support and he was always there for us.

He had so many responsibilities and yet he never complained.'

The news is grim. All of us know that Mr El-Hawrani will not be the last of us to die. As in Italy, where coronavirus has already killed fifty doctors, this is only the beginning. The chair of the British Medical Association, Dr Chaand Nagpaul, responds to the Italian medical death toll by writing: 'It is with deep sadness and horror that we learn that the lives of more than 50 doctors have now been lost in Italy to Covid-19 ... British doctors have looked to Italy with trepidation as the spread here continues, as we are naturally concerned that we may face a challenge of the same scale within weeks. The bravery and compassion shown by our Italian colleagues in the most harrowing circumstances is an inspiration to us.'

He is wrong, though. There is nothing inspiring about these doctors' deaths, nor those of nurses, paramedics, porters, cleaners or any of the other frontline staff who put their lives at risk by doing their jobs. My heart quails as I think of the medical students volunteering so eagerly, without hesitation. And of the retired clinicians who, despite knowing that their age makes them particularly vulnerable to Covid, have volun-teered in their thousands to return to NHS service. Already, the government has enthusiastically taken to describing us all as 'heroes'. But accolades will not keep anyone safe. For that, we need proper PPE.

Just a few days prior to Mr El-Hawrani's death, the British Medical Association issued a blunt public warning to the gov-ernment. Without enough PPE, the BMA predicted, doctors were going to die. Frontline staff, they reported, were being forced to buy their own protective equipment from high-street DIY chains or to cobble together homemade kit amid widespread shortages of PPE in hospitals, GP surgeries and care homes. Nagpaul described growing evidence that 'thousands of GPs and hospital staff are still not being provided with the kit they need to properly protect themselves and their patients . . . We are being asked to risk our lives, and our loved ones' lives, in flimsy paper masks and plastic aprons. I just don't know if I can. I don't think it is fair to expect this of us. I am terrified. How can this risk to practitioners, other patients, practitioners' families be justified?'

Nagpaul's words have been echoed all week on social media by hundreds of nurses, carers, paramedics and other allied health professionals. Even *after* PPE standards had been downgraded for the majority of frontline staff, the appropriate kit was still unavailable for many of them. Three nurses from the recently overwhelmed Northwick Park Hospital in London shared a photo of themselves with bin bags on their heads and feet as they issued a plea for proper masks, gowns and gloves. They told the *Daily Telegraph* they had had to 'use their initiative' by wearing the bin liners, as they had 'no other choice' due to the lack of PPE available. Shortly afterwards, all three nurses test positive for Covid.

Social media takes on a feverish quality as our incredulity burns. Phrases like 'cannon fodder' and 'lambs to the slaughter' scorch Facebook and Twitter, and rightly so. My stomach turns at the thought of a wealthy country sending out its nurses to face Covid in bin bags. As Nagpaul puts it: 'A construction worker wouldn't be allowed to work without a hard hat and proper boots. Even a bee-keeper wouldn't inspect a hive without proper protective clothing. And yet this government expects NHS staff to put themselves at risk of serious illness, or even death, by treating highly infectious Covid-19 patients without wearing proper protection. This is totally unacceptable.'

The government tries to sidestep the issue by describing the millions of pieces of PPE they are sending out, as if this somehow airbrushes out of existence the first-hand testimony from frontline staff. Later, to the incandescent rage of doctors and nurses, it transpires that the government boosted its numbers by counting the individual gloves in one pair as *two* separate items of kit. Meanwhile, Alan Hoskins, the chief officer of the Health Care Supply Association, takes to Twitter in sheer desperation after being unable to order PPE, even having escalated the matter to NHS England. His tweet, which he subsequently deletes, states: 'What a day, no gowns in NHS Supply Chain. Rang every number escalated to NHS England, just got message back – no stock, can't help, can send you a PPE pack. Losing the will to live, God help us all.'

The same day, my brother-in-law, a former teacher, sends me a message to say that members of his local Scouts Association are making visors in their back gardens and that he will send us some as soon as he can. Locked-down children, it turns out, are stepping in to supply the NHS with PPE where the government has failed. God help us all indeed.

On the last day of March, Laura Wood sits down at her mum's kitchen table and starts writing in a spiral-bound notebook. 'Dear Dad, I thought it might be nice for you if we kept a diary whilst you've been so unwell. Just so that when you are back home you can make sense of everything that's happened while you've been in hospital.'

Her father, Ken, has been in ICU for twenty-four hours and

Laura is being more than a thoughtful daughter. As an ICU nurse, she knows how precious these diaries, written in snatches of calm by the nurses who know their patients so intimately, can be. If you set out to design the most deliberately disorientating environment imaginable, you could do worse than mimic an ICU with its flashing and bleeping, its space-age machinery, its parade of alien faces in identikit scrubs, and the cocktails of mind-altering drugs that course through each patient's veins. With Covid, even the anchoring humanity of faces is gone. Masks and hoods, not people, dip and weave above your bed. Small wonder that when a patient wakes up, they are often delirious.

Should a patient emerge from an ICU coma with demons and devils crowding their brains, a patient diary can be a vital counterpoint to their hallucinatory haze, an alternative reality based in fact, not psychosis. And for those patients who are destined never to resurface, Laura knows that these handwritten records, invariably brimming with affection and detail, give grieving relatives a testament of tenderness that may help frame their loss. Alongside the drugs and drama of critical illness, they speak of brushed teeth, scented hand cream, whispered silliness, smoothed hair. Yes, he was here, a diary will tell you – amid all the jangling and machinery and the endless tubes – but he was loved, he was human, he was a person who mattered, and we enfolded him within our care.

'That night,' Laura writes to her father, 'you went from A&E to the ward. But during the night you needed more oxygen than they can give. So they moved you on to the intensive care unit. At first, they put you on an oxygen therapy called nasal high flow. This can give higher percentages of oxygen but this still wasn't enough and you needed even more. At this point your lungs which have been working so hard for so long started to wilt/sag so they needed some pressure to blow them up again properly. This is when they will have put that horrible mask on you. I can imagine you felt quite awful at this point. Despite all of this your body was just getting so tired and the consultant decided it was time for you to be put to sleep and let a ventilator take over all the hard work you've been doing.'

With every word she writes – this meticulous committing of her father's story to paper – fear sits like a stone on Laura's chest. She must maintain an absolute conviction that he *will* read these words. If she allows herself to consider the alternative, even for an instant, her hand trembles too much to write. He *will* walk through this front door, Bertie the dog *will* fling himself madly at Dad's unsteady legs, and life *will* resume where it stopped so abruptly, curtailed by a virus that, though mindless, is deadly.

The kitchen Laura sits in is bursting with flowers, the freezer filled with homemade meals from thoughtful neighbours desperate to help. Ken is a man of deep faith and the whole family have been cocooned within the extravagant kindness of church, friends and neighbours, no gesture, no offer of help too much. Laura bites her lip in concentration. She will not splinter, she will cling to her hope. It is an act of faith that takes all she has, but she continues, painstakingly, to write: 'Dad, you wouldn't even believe the amount of love and support everyone has shown to the whole family through all of this. Everyone we know is praying for you. It just shows what a wonderful father and man you are. We love you so, so much. We are all just so heartbroken this is happening to you. I really wish you could see all the love there is out here for you, Dad. You are going to get through this.'

7

Inside the Wave

*I sit, slack-jawed . . . at history's unfolding . . . The names
of the dead, the shock at their number and improbability, the
forecasts for the future, the dismal withdrawal and isolation,
left one, in the end, speechless. Impotent.*

ANDREW HOLLERAN, *Chronicle of a Plague,
Revisited: AIDS and Its Aftermath*

Albert Jenkins was born the same year that Britain and France
declared war on Germany. I smile involuntarily when his granddaughter tells me this, thinking briefly of my own grandparents,
both long deceased, who were married on the very day that
World War Two broke out, 3 September 1939. At 11.15 a.m.
precisely that Sunday, Prime Minister Neville Chamberlain
broke the news to the nation in a radio address from the Cabinet
Room in 10 Downing Street. An hour later, having been
granted emergency dispensation by an obliging chaplain for a
Sunday wedding, my grandparents were hastily married. Shortly
after that, as the first barrage balloons went up over London,

Granny – then in her twenties – was tipsy on green chartreuse in an East End pub with her new husband. A few days later, he was sent to sea, a naval doctor who would spend most of the next five years playing cat-and-mouse with U-boats in the north Atlantic. (My father, my grandfather and even my great-grandfather were physicians: medicine is in my blood.)

Albie, as he likes to be known, has traversed eight decades in remarkably good health. Apart from a surgeon removing his rotting appendix during childhood – the NHS would have been in its infancy then – he has never needed a hospital. His daughter lost her life to cancer in her sixties and yet Albie, for all the pleasure he had taken in Woodbines and strong bitter, carried on. Now, he has been admitted with coronavirus and I am speaking on the phone to his next-of-kin, his granddaughter Christine. 'Tell me about him,' I've just asked. 'What does he enjoy? What kind of man is he?' Any details I can glean may help build a rapport with my patient that reaches beyond my visor and mask. Equally, I am hoping my questions may convey to Christine that though her grandfather is sequestered away in the hospital, to us he is someone who matters. The absent agony of relatives, I am learning, is the pandemic's cruellest feature.

The Covid ward is humid and restive. We are on the move, no pausing or lingering, with strained expressions and a twitchy hypervigilance that is as exhausting and stifling as the masks we wear. It is all around us, the virus. It coats our clothes, our hair, the backs of our necks, the keyboards we type on, the surfaces we touch. It hangs in the air, it drops on to our shoes, it floats and waits, ready to be inhaled by anyone too unwell to be masked up in a hot zone. Someone, that is, like a patient. For what unites the men and women on this ward – whether suspected or known to have Covid – is how very vulnerable they are. Most are too ill or too agitated to tolerate a protective mask. Trying to impose one is at best futile, at worst downright cruel, with patients who are delirious, distressed or suffering from severe dementia. Tangled lines and tubes and masks can be intolerably alien to them. I have seen disorientated patients ripping oxygen masks off their faces, cannulas from their veins and even, with the catheter balloon fully inflated, catheters straight out of their bladders.

Ideally, of course, we would protect every patient by rigidly segregating the infected from the non-infected. But how? How can we do this when Covid tests are currently taking four or more days to come back from a laboratory, yet new patients pour into A&E every hour? As it stands in early April, the UK's pitiful testing capacity, when compared to similar European countries like Germany, makes a mockery of the red and blue zones which the hospital moved mountains to create in days. By definition, we cannot separate Covid from non-Covid until we know which is which. Yet in the days it takes for a test to be turned around, a single patient could have infected the rest of their ward. I choke down a sudden surge of bitterness and anger. Hasn't the government had since *January* to prepare for this? How can we possibly have abandoned all attempts to test patients in community settings, yet *still* have insufficient capacity for prompt testing of patients and staff in hospital?

Hunched over a phone at the back of the nurses' station, I strain to catch Christine's words against the thrum of the ward. Albie was brought by ambulance from his home, a small terraced cottage on the edge of town, to the hospital two nights ago. Christine's apologies tumble so fast from her mouth I can hardly make out what she's saying. 'The advice was to shield, so I didn't dare visit. But I spoke to him every day. He always said he was fine. But yesterday he just seemed odd. He never likes to complain. When he said he wasn't breathing properly, well, I just knew it was bad. I called 999 straight away. But I should have called sooner. Or visited him. I should have visited. Why didn't I visit?'

Above the static and crackle of the ward around me, guilt spills out of the phone. Christine's words are laced with self-recrimination. At eighty, Albie has been dutifully avoiding all contact with others. Christine too has slavishly obeyed government advice to protect her closest family from harm, dropping a bag of groceries on his doorstep twice a week, ordering him overpriced alcohol gel online, and phoning daily to check up on him. Despite it all, now he is fighting for his life, alone in a hospital, with some disembodied doctor she can't even see saying she's so sorry, but he is 'sick enough to die'.

In normal times, I would be sitting side by side with Christine, alert to every visual nuance – perhaps a creasing of brows, a whitening of knuckles, a twitch of the muscles at the angle of her jaw as it clenches. And, if I managed to do my job well, she might read in turn from my facial expression that there is no shame, she has not failed, she has done everything possible, but this disease is implacable. As it is, the new normal – a phrase I have come to detest – dictates what is possible. I can barely hear her words and mine are so muffled behind my mask that twice she has to ask me to speak louder. It is grotesque, a parody of communication. It could not be less warm, more wrong.

'Christine, would you like to come and visit your grandfather?'

I semi-shout into the receiver. 'You would need to wear PPE but we can show you how to put it on, and you can be with him in his room.'

'I thought that wasn't allowed? No visitors?'

'Usually that's right,' I explain, 'but because we believe his time is so short now, you can absolutely come in and visit Albie.'

I am hoping Christine will clutch at this straw, find a chink of relief in being able to be with her grandfather. But the pause is long and her words fall like stones. 'Will – that's my husband – is shielding. He's on chemo. He has bowel cancer.'

It takes me a moment to compute what this means. Were Christine to visit her dying grandfather, she might bring back home, straight to Will and his battered immune system, the very thing that is wresting her grandfather's life from him. Her visit, in short, could be the death of her husband.

Lockdown. Covid has this woman checkmated.

'I – I need to talk to Will,' Christine mutters.

We agree she will call back shortly and I realise my fingers have tightened around a sheet of paper, as if by crumpling its edges I might obliterate the words I've scrawled. Albie's, you see, is only the first name on my list. There are more just like him to attend to. A handwritten tally of today's pandemic casualties. I grit my teeth. My colleague and I are immersed in something both momentous and terrible. We have never been here before. Death has been daily news for so long now I am beginning to feel like a plague doctor.

In this radically rearranged world, the hospital is unrecognisable. Everything inessential has been ruthlessly suspended, with staff dispatched to the red zones that so desperately need them: A&E, acute medicine, intensive care. Overnight, whole wards, whole floors, have essentially been mothballed. Hip replacements, cataract removals, cardiac scans, liver biopsies – all too much of this vital activity is history. Clinical wastelands separate frenetic islands of activity from one another. Visitors are largely banished.

In A&E, patients with suspected Covid are sifted and streamed so treatments can be tailored to individuals. Patients may end up in one of three different locations. Some wards, like Albie's, do not carry out any of the procedures such as CPAP that require the highest levels of PPE. Patients here are so frail or weak that anything more invasive than simple oxygen and intravenous drugs has been judged to have harmful effects that are likely to outweigh the benefits. Then there are other Covid wards on which the doctors may intervene more aggressively. Devices, such as CPAP, that enable the delivery of a higher concentration of oxygen are used if the patient is sufficiently robust to withstand them. Lastly, the most extreme interventions occur in intensive care. Here, if CPAP can no longer prevent a patient's lungs from failing, they may be intubated and connected to a ventilator. Occasionally, when even a ventilator cannot supply a patient with sufficient oxygen, they may be transported to a specialist centre to be connected to a machine for extra-corporeal membrane oxygenation. In ECMO, rather than extra oxygen being forced from outside into the lungs, the patient's blood is pumped out of their body and through a machine that externally oxygenates it. It is the mechanical equivalent of a pair of human lungs in a fish tank.

Nowhere is more oppressive or more gruelling for staff than the intensive care unit. In the wider hospital community, we are fiercely proud of our ICU colleagues who, without exception, refuse to acknowledge that they are doing anything special at all. Chris Acott, an ICU registrar, cared for his first Covid patient in the ICU in early March. 'Back then,' he tells me, 'I wasn't scared at all. I had that superficial arrogance of being a clinician. I thought, Well, this is straightforward single organ failure. I've got this, this is my bag.'

It did not take long working in the 'Covid pit', as ICU staff quickly christened it, for Chris to revise his opinion. 'By the end of my second or third day I was thinking, My God, actually this is really bad. I went completely the opposite way. I started telling my friends and family, "No, listen, this is bad, this is serious. Don't listen to the government. Only go out if you need the essentials."'

What transformed Chris's complacency was how exceptionally sick the Covid patients he was treating were. 'Secretly, I'd initially thought, Well, I'm young and healthy so if I do get it, I'll probably be fine. But we started hearing about people around the country who were equally young and fit, yet still died. Then, we admitted someone to our ICU who was essentially healthy, in their early thirties, with minimal co-morbidities. I'm twenty-nine. That brought it home. This could be any of us.' He pauses. 'And of course, I lost some of my faith in the PPE when we started admitting staff members. There was a lot of fear among my nursing and medical colleagues. It rubs off. It all melds together into one soup of stress, anxiety and uncertainty.'

Long before lockdown, based on everything he witnessed, Chris avoided his own family and advised them to stay at home whenever possible. 'I was most worried about infecting my wife and also my niece and my pregnant sister-in-law. Much more pressing though was Poppy, my littlest sister, who had just turned eight and has cystic fibrosis.' Poppy's lung condition leaves her exceptionally vulnerable to any form of pneumonia, let alone a condition as severe as Covid. Her mother and sisters were able to follow Chris's advice and shield at home with Poppy. But her father, a community pharmacy manager, was the family breadwinner. 'He is the only person who earns money in the household, so he had to go to work,' Chris explains. 'There was no alternative. That obviously put Poppy at risk, which Dad couldn't accept. So he got an old mattress, stuck it in the garage, tried to seal up the draught underneath the garage door and has lived there ever since, sleeping with the tools, the washing machine, the junk and the old cardboard boxes. If you want an example of a family who have been hit hardest by lockdown without getting Covid, they are it. Dad's been in social isolation from the rest of his entire family, only talking to them on the phone, only seeing his wife and children through the windows. It takes extreme self-control and I am not sure I would have the strength to do it. I have the utmost respect for him.'

Chris's father will go on to spend four whole months alone on that mattress in his garage, showering at work, eating in isolation, with only a laptop for company. Such is his fear of endangering his daughter, such is his resolve to protect her. And it is like this now all across the country, for all but the most reckless individuals. Behind closed doors, unheard, unnoticed – these clandestine acts of love and sacrifice, too multitudinous to count.

*

The ICU is drenched in Covid. From the throats and hearts and lungs of the patients who lie faceless on their fronts, somewhere in the space between lying and dying, the virus blooms and lingers. The cleaners, physiotherapists, dieticians, nurses, carers and doctors who work in the unit all do so while endeavouring to manage the fear of becoming infected themselves. You have no choice, the patients need you. But like everything else with this disease, the effectiveness of the PPE you wear is unknown and untested. You brace yourself for the worst.

As one of only a handful of junior doctors with independent airway skills – the ability to intubate patients without supervision – Chris swiftly becomes a predominantly 'in-pit' doctor. Entering the pit entails the rigmarole of protecting himself with the highest level of PPE: rubber boots, a full-length surgical gown, a respirator hood, a plastic apron and no fewer than three sets of gloves. A scrappy sign in the PPE room reads 'Pee before you PPE'. The kit, however, is no laughing matter. 'Once you get over the sudden increase in body temperature, the fact that you can't really breathe, that you're tripping over your feet and that you can't feel anything any more in your fingers, it gets more tolerable with time,' says Chris, 'but everything about PPE makes it harder to do your job and more likely that you will make a mistake. People don't realise how hard it is to breathe. It's as though you're face down on your bed, the duvet's over your head and you're trying to breathe with a pillow pressed on to your face – for hours at a time.'

The masks worn in ICU are not only claustrophobic and suffocating, they dig deeply into the flesh along the bridge of the nose and cheekbones, causing harsh indentations. Doctors and nurses take to wearing strips of surgical tape across their noses in an effort to protect their skin from breaking down. Some develop abrasions and even ulcerations, their skin chafed and weeping. Yet what hurts staff most about the pit is not its physical demands, but the psychological assault of seeing patients so entirely cut off from their loved ones. 'Usually, there are cards, drinks, photos, blankets — all these little signs of normality, of humanity, that patients' relatives bring to the unit,' Chris tells me. 'Without visitors and the gifts they bring, the ICU feels like a laboratory or a machine, focused on supporting numbers in beds, not people.'

I try to conjure this dystopian world from a patient's perspective. Touching, holding and embracing — those quintessential human acts — are forbidden. Doctors bellow to make themselves heard. Days and weeks pass and in all that time you do not see a single unmasked human face, no lips, no cheeks, no smiles.

In the pit, beds have been crammed into every spare corner to make space for those in need. 'Patients are almost shoulder to shoulder,' Chris says. The physical proximity forces an intimacy of the most harrowing kind. Patients sometimes find themselves unwilling onlookers as a neighbour's lungs give out for the last time. 'When that happens, which it does, I can only imagine they must lie there fearing they are watching themselves in the future,' says Chris. 'It is the most traumatic thing imaginable, people stuck in rooms looking at other people who are dying of exactly the same disease.'

Take the hi-tech equipment away and this is the stuff of battlefield triage, the living and dying side by side. Chris hesitates before speaking of what keeps him going. 'There is no way to over-exaggerate how wonderful the staff around me are and how caring and loving they have been. The nurses especially are the surrogate family for the people who needed them most. They care so much. You have no idea. And it is so heartening to see. Despite the chronic NHS underfunding, with staff retention at an all-time low, when we don't have enough people, when we've got more clinical demands on us than ever before – still the nurses and everyone else manage to find the time to keep caring. That is a beautiful thing and I hope we never lose it.'

Alice Warwick, twenty-seven, has been the deputy sister on the adult ICU for a little over two years. She has the fine features, blonde hair and slender frame that might make a certain kind of man infer fragility – though if they did, they could not be more wrong. Alice is one of the most resilient people I have ever met. There is no one you would rather have by your side in a crisis. Indeed, crisis is her natural habitat. On the unit, every one of her patients is critical. Having reached the absolute limit of what a human frame can withstand, they pivot between death and recovery. Most people would run a mile from such high stakes. Alice, Chris and their ICU colleagues are drawn to them. But even here, Covid stands out.

'The virus follows no rules – it is something else,' she tells me. 'The slightest of movements can destabilise a Covid patient. They can crash, desaturate, and it will take you half an hour to recover them.'

During her shifts in the Covid pit, Alice leads the small team of nurses caring for the patients in one bay. Normally – that word again – ICU patients are so severely unwell they require 1:1 nursing. A nurse's twelve-hour shift is devoted to one patient alone – they receive the best of you, all you have. Now though, perhaps six nurses are responsible for eight patients, with only three of them having had any training in intensive care. The team is too sparse, stretched twice as thinly as normal, and every patient is as sick as any Alice has known.

'At the peak, they'd arrive one after the other, all in respiratory failure. They'd need two or three nurses and two doctors to stabilise them. They were on a knife edge. You'd sort one, then go on to the next one. It's undignified, a conveyor belt, but there's nothing else you can do. You are running on adrenalin.'

Each bay of patients is sealed to contain its viral load. The only way to communicate with the outside world is through telephones, one in each bay, with which members of the nursing team must call for more suction, more oxygen, the back-up of a doctor, senior help. In the early days, to try to contain the contagion the nurses found the bays had been over-zealously stripped of extraneous equipment. Running out of essentials mid-crisis was common and they learned on the job to squeeze in more kit.

'I assumed I'd get it,' Alice tells me. 'How could you *not* bring the virus out of an environment like that? It's so crammed, so busy, everyone so close together. In your PPE you can't hear properly, you can't see properly, you can't be heard properly and patients are deteriorating all around you. It feels a bit like a war zone.'

Each ventilator delivers its breaths like a metronome, the patients' chests rising and falling with perfect regularity. Two seconds in, two seconds out, the timing, pressure and depth of each enforced inhalation titrated to match the extent to which Covid has ravaged these lungs. At any one time, the nurses may be fine-tuning the doses of drugs in six or more separate infusions that feed into a central line in a patient's neck. The team are discovering that after the lungs fail, Covid can quickly cripple the kidneys and heart as well. 'They are cardiovascularly unstable, on inotropes to try and maintain their blood pressure, and we are constantly tweaking to try and keep their pressures stable. The patients are teetering on the brink, all at the same time. But there's only one of you. It's exhausting.' The hardest thing of all, Alice goes on to tell me, is seeing so many critically unwell patients 'lined up like bodies' in the bay. Often, being prone, the patients' faces are hidden. 'No faces. No relatives. No personal details. People are stripped of their life and their character. Everything human has been taken away.'

Covid even steals the patients' names. So great are the risks of miscommunication in PPE that it is safer for the nursing team to use bed numbers to refer to the human beings for whom they care. Covid, in short, necessarily compromises every instinct to deliver humane and compassionate care. It violates something at the heart of good medicine – and the cost to the team is profound. For the first time in her life, Alice has begun talking in her sleep. Soon she is sleepwalking through the house at night. Spiders stalk her dreams, whose nightmarish quality is triggered by conditions at work she has never endured before. For a time, Alice quietly tells me, 'coronavirus took my hardiness away'.

There is a concept in healthcare which perhaps underpins the ICU team's feelings of derailment. The term 'moral injury' was first used to describe soldiers' psychological responses to their actions in war. 'Potentially morally injurious events, such as perpetrating, failing to prevent, or bearing witness to acts that transgress deeply held moral beliefs and expectations, may be deleterious in the long-term, emotionally, psychologically, behaviourally, spiritually, and socially,' states a 2009 paper in the *Clinical Psychology Review*. In healthcare, the crux of moral injury is a practitioner's sense that they are failing consistently to meet their patients' needs, often due to systemic factors beyond their control such as, in this case, the dehumanising consequences of rigorous infection control. The sense of complicity in providing inadequate or inhumane care can lead to well-documented feelings of guilt and anguish.

There is one saving grace amid the pain of the pit. Whatever Covid takes, no matter how it distorts their usual care, the team are resolved that no one in their unit will die alone. They will not permit the virus that. Sometimes, at the end, it may be Alice who sits at a patient's bedside. Always, without fail, a member of staff will be there. Above the suck and the hiss of the machines, amid the technological detritus of intensive care, someone will clasp a hand, whisper words of comfort, read messages of love from family members out loud, and sit and wait until life is extinguished.

On the general wards of the hospital, as in the ICU, staff are learning, in fits and starts, how to mitigate the cruelties a pandemic bestows. 'I've got a plan,' announces Mandi with conspiratorial glee. Mandi Kitching is a specialist palliative care nurse and her plans, without fail, have her patients at their heart. With her multiple piercings and feisty demeanour, you could easily feel a little intimidated by Mandi. Her devotion to her patients is fierce.

'Go on,' I grin. 'What are you plotting?'

'Well. It's about Albert Jenkins. If Christine can't come to him, let's bring him to Christine.'

I raise an eyebrow. Mandi, it turns out, has procured an iPad from somewhere. For all I know, she might have raided the trust CEO's office. She would think nothing of liberating a piece of kit for someone who needs it.

We walk together to Albie's room and Mandi prepares to call Christine. He has the same greyish pallor I'd observed earlier, his chest rising and falling erratically – a sign that death may be drawing near. Something is different, however. I look more closely. It is not just that our drugs have helped relax and soothe him. Mandi, I realise, has washed Albie's face and neatly combed his hair. 'I talked to him the whole time while I was doing it,' she tells me. 'I told him how much Christine loved him.' In managerial spreadsheets of what counts as value, there is no column, no row, for these actions of Mandi's. The vocabulary of efficiency, productivity, growth and profit makes a mockery of the time she has spent in this room – the words she whispered unheard to a dying man, the hands she laid unfelt upon his cheeks and brow. But if a language erases what cannot be counted, then it is broken, unfit for purpose. For what Mandi has given of herself at Albie's bedside – this unchecked flow of love and care – is both intangible and priceless. Because here now is Christine, crackling into life on an iPad of dubious provenance, and through her tears I hear her say, 'Gramps, don't you look smart!' as Mandi tilts the screen so that Albie's face, these unfocused eyes, this precise side-parting, fill the centre of his granddaughter's frame of vision.

Christine talks and talks, as though Albie is hanging upon every word, as though if she stopped she might never start again. Finally, she goes quiet as she fiddles with the buttons on her phone, then makes a little announcement. 'Remember how you and Gran would go courting, Gramps? The dances you told me about? Here you are, Gramps. Here's a bit of Buddy Holly.'

In the hospice we are preparing to admit our first patients with Covid – our beds newly expanded from ten to twenty-six – when Charlie, the medical director, asks me into his office for a quiet word. 'We have a problem,' he tells me. 'We don't have anything like enough PPE.'

A new government directive has just been issued. In the eyes of many clinicians, it is at least several weeks too late. Nevertheless, the new rule is here: anyone who works within two metres of patients, irrespective of whether a patient is suspected of infection with Covid, must wear Level 1 PPE. At a minimum, this constitutes a fluid-resistant paper mask, an apron, gloves and, if the risk of splashes is significant, a visor too. The revised guidance is entirely right. Sustained community transmission of Covid is now well established and has probably been so for some time. Any one of our patients may therefore be infected and no one working in clinical areas should be put at risk of contracting a potentially fatal disease through lack of PPE.

There is just one snag with the guidance (which, I note, still falls short of the WHO's minimum standards). Any non-hospital clinical setting – be that a care home, a general practice or a hospice – has been issued with the same standard PPE pack. It contains a roll of plastic aprons, some gloves and a box of 300 paper face masks, some of which have a best-before date of 2016. To put the inadequacy of these supplies into sharp relief, at the Katharine House Response Centre we are estimating a *daily* requirement of at least 150 masks. Thus, at precisely the same time as we are reconfiguring the entire hospice at break-neck speed to admit patients dying of Covid, the government has provided us with a stock of masks that will last, at most, for two days. You might as well push a passenger out of a plane with a handkerchief in lieu of a parachute.

'What about the emergency PPE line?' I ask Charlie in confusion. 'Haven't they been able to sort it?' After the slew of negative headlines about desperate NHS staff using bin bags, homemade visors and builders' masks for protection, the government has hastily announced a new 24/7 emergency NHS Supply Chain hotline. This, we have been assured with much public fanfare, will enable any health or care teams in crisis to obtain urgent supplies of PPE. Naively, I'd imagined some kind of superhero hybrid of Matt Hancock and the bat phone – one call and a caped crusader would instantly swoop to our rescue.

The reality is jarring. 'We've been calling and emailing the Supply Chain all week,' Charlie tells me. 'Multiple times. You leave messages, no one calls you back, it's a disaster.' Today is Wednesday. The hospice has managed to augment our tiny stock of masks by begging extras from generous local builders and veterinary practices, but at this rate we will run out completely on Friday. And we are not alone. On Twitter, I see, some of London's largest hospices are also posting plaintive appeals for masks and aprons. St Joseph's Hospice in Hackney tweets: 'URGENT APPEAL – Our frontline staff are working 24 hours a day to ensure that our patients receive the very best care. But we're still without PPE. Please, please provide us with SFP3 [sic] masks, long gowns, gloves, plastic aprons and sanitiser gel so that we can work safely.'

Charlie is a man of great gentleness and decency but even he can barely contain his rage. 'Eventually I managed to speak to someone, but they told me there was nothing they could do. I insisted that wasn't good enough. I said I was the medical director of a hospice which was twenty-four hours away from having to close all its beds and discharge its inpatients if we could not get more masks. They weren't interested. They just gave me another number at the Department of Health to call, but there was no answer and I went through to another machine. What do I do?' He raises his palms wide as if to summon an answer from the air as we stare at each other across the room.

I'm so angry, I can scarcely breathe. Tears sting at the corners of my eyes. 'Can I make sure I have understood this accurately?' I say to Charlie, endeavouring to keep my voice level. 'If we cannot get a delivery of masks tomorrow for the staff to wear – basic paper masks – we are going to have to close the hospice and send all our patients away? Some of whom are actively dying, in the final days or even hours of their lives?' He nods helplessly. 'And the response to this, from the official emergency PPE hotline, was, No, sorry, there is nothing we can do to help you?'

He nods again, and I stare at my shoes. So this is how our society has decided to treat its most vulnerable members. The government's rapidly constructed pandemic narrative invokes 'heroism', the 'Blitz spirit', the country 'coming together' and yet, in all this noise and bellicose playacting, it seems the residents of hospices have been forgotten, abandoned, as they quietly approach the end of their lives, facing eviction for want of some paper masks.

I look up. 'I will fix this,' I tell Charlie, trying to keep my voice steady. 'I don't know how but I will get us the masks we need.'

I send a message to a friend and colleague. Like me, Dominic

Pimenta, a London-based doctor who specialises in cardiology, has been aghast at the sluggishness with which lockdown, testing and the provision of PPE have been addressed over the last two months. Remarkably, alongside his clinical workload as a junior doctor redeployed to a Covid ICU, Dom has set up a charity called HEROES aimed at protecting and supporting health and care workers. The response from the public has been overwhelmingly positive and, in a matter of weeks, Dom's charity has raised over a million pounds. It is an extraordinary achievement. If anyone can help my hospice inpatients, he can. My message is distraught:

> Dear Dom, I'm sorry to bother you when you are probably 1,000% too busy, but I am desperate . . . My hospice is on the brink of having to close the entire inpatient unit because we cannot get surgical masks from anywhere. We've tried the emergency NHS Covid supply chain people, even tried all our local vets, but the NHS aren't helping us and we can't keep staff and patients safe so may have to close completely by this weekend. I'm not sure if you have funds for PPE, but can I possibly beg for some masks? Just asking out of sheer desperation.

Dom's reply is terse: 'I'll see what we can do.'

I try not to feel too crestfallen. I am absolutely certain he will help if he can and attribute his caution to avoiding raising my hopes prematurely. That evening, though, I am distracted. 'You keep looking at your phone more than us,' complains an indignant Abbey. I creep away, too restless to focus on my husband and children – an occurrence far too common of late.

Even if I do manage to find some masks for Katharine House, the UK has another 220 independent hospices. There must be hundreds more terminally ill patients at precisely the same risk as ours of being turfed from their beds and out of their hospices to go – who knows where? And who, apparently, even cares?

Most uncomfortably of all, I consider the significance of the fact that in government supply chain terms, hospices are the lowest priority for PPE because we are classified not as hospitals but as care homes. In the UK, there are over 400,000 elderly and disabled people living in care homes. These are precisely the people most at risk of dying from Covid, the people we are meant to be doing our utmost to shield. I think back to the words of Patrick Vallance, the government's Chief Scientific Adviser, when he stood on a podium alongside Boris Johnson in early March and assured the watching press and public that 'Central to all of this is making sure that we protect the vulnerable. The highest-risk groups are the elderly and those with pre-existing illnesses, and those are the ones we've got to take most care to protect during this.'

If those really were the intentions, how has it come to this, a month later, that each of the nation's 30,000 care homes has been given nothing more than a two-day supply of masks apiece, forcing upon staff the impossible choice of abandoning their residents or going to work unprotected? I understand and agree that if PPE is scarce it should be conserved for our colleagues in the highest-risk areas. But to pretend, as the government is doing, that there is sufficient PPE to go around is spectacularly dishonest. Staff are scrambling to do the best we can with what we have. But the reality is we do not have enough, our best is barely up to scratch, patients and staff are

being endangered – and we have had since January to pro-
cure the PPE that should, even now, be protecting 400,000 of
Britain's most vulnerable citizens from a virus we have known
all along may kill them.

When my phone rings, a number I do not recognise, I lunge
for it. Dom has indeed – *you absolute legend* – been quietly at
work behind the scenes, talking to a man called Paul Ford from
the Contractors Appeal, another charity set up to supply the
NHS and carers with much-needed PPE. 'I've sorted it,' Paul
tells me. 'We will deliver a thousand masks to your hospice
tomorrow morning.'

To Paul's considerable discomfort, he is forced to listen to
a semi-hysterical palliative care doctor sobbing her heartfelt
thanks down the phone at him. Immediately I message Charlie
to tell him the good news, and then Dom who, alongside Paul,
has achieved something truly wonderful: 'Dom!!! Paul can
deliver 1000 masks tomorrow. I literally burst into tears on the
phone. I cannot tell you how grateful we all are – just thank
you, a million times.'

Our patients, at least temporarily, are safe. Thanks to the
public's entrepreneurial and charitable instincts, a hospice will
remain open this weekend when it might otherwise have been
forced to close its doors. But I pace the kitchen that night, brain
jangling. The wrongness of it all makes my heart pound. It is
abundantly clear that our patients were no one's priority. No
one in power had properly considered them. There is a hierarchy to dying, as with everything else, and those approaching
the end of their lives, whether through extremes of age or a
life-limiting illness, are evidently at the bottom. I think of the
Albies, the Winstons and all the others I am treating in the

twilight of their lives who may be frail and weary – who may even have lived through the war now invoked by politicians so lightly – yet whose end should most definitely not be now. And I lay my head on my arms and weep in the dark for all the things I cannot do and all the death there has been and is yet to come.

8

The Thing with Feathers

There is a crack in everything, that's how the light gets in.

LEONARD COHEN, 'Anthem'

In a small terraced house on the edge of Banbury sits a woman on a sofa beside a ball of red wool, her fingers darting as swiftly and deftly as a chime of wrens. Like many of us now, in the thick of the pandemic, Sandra is frightened. Everything has been upended. A trip to the supermarket entails queuing for hours and once inside, all the flour and yeast will be gone, as though the country intends to bake its way out of the crisis. Dangers lurk unseen in the world beyond her doorstep. One false move, one reckless inhalation and the virus could be there, in your lungs, proliferating. Sandra paces and frets and disinfects surfaces as she tries to keep her anxieties at bay. Each day the news announces a world more frightening than the day before. We shiver with dread and try to manage the fear of losing those we love, or of them losing us. Lockdown is life interrupted.

One day, Sandra finds herself rummaging in her wool basket, unsure of what she intends to find. It is her sixtieth birthday and, as she considers her good fortune to have arrived at this age, she feels propelled to do something for others. She thinks of her local hospital, the Horton General, and all that the patients and staff must be going through there. An idea begins to form.

She pulls out a ball the colour of blood, drawn to the richness of crimson. She takes her crochet hook in one hand, settles down by the window and begins methodically, almost rhythmically, to braid a miniature of the one thing she is certain matters more than anything in these times of tumult and loss. In the hour it takes her to craft the tiny symbol, her mind flutters less distractingly and her breathing slows. She looks down at the splash of redness nestled in her palms and, for the first time that morning, she smiles. This little woollen metaphor – a heart that spans no more than an inch – has both calmed her nerves and inspired a manifesto for action.

'Dear Everyone in the NHS,' Sandra writes later that day. 'Thank you with all my HEARTS for everything you are doing to keep us safe and alive, so that when we meet up with our loved ones once more, no one is missing. You are our NHS angels. Love and blessings, Sandra.'

Sandra has decided she will work and work until she has stuffed a Jiffy bag with sixty crocheted hearts – one for each year of her life – and deliver them to the Horton. When her package is opened by the hospital receptionist, she immediately picks up her phone and calls Mandi Kitching. If anyone would know where Sandra's gifts are needed most, it is a specialist palliative care nurse. And so one day, a bag of hearts appears on the desk of my pierced, peroxided partner in crime, who immediately conceives a plan of brilliance.

What proliferates in a pandemic, it turns out, takes human as well as viral form. Suddenly, small acts of kindness like Sandra's are rife. Yes, there are the frantic toilet-roll hoarders who ransack supermarket shelves until their car boots are bulging. And yes, in London, briefly and incredibly, junior doctors are mugged for their NHS ID badges so that some cheapskate assailant can purloin a free high-street coffee intended for NHS staff. There will always be the grifters, the freeloaders, the exploiters. But by and large, something extraordinary is underway. Spontaneously, impulsively, house by house, hour by hour, a street revolution is sweeping the country.

At first, I'm so immersed in my clinical work that this groundswell of caring almost passes me by. One evening I pull into my village and blink in astonishment. Rainbows have sprung up in all the neighbours' windows, gorgeous in their gaudiness and wonky messages of thanks. Children paint 'We love our key workers!' and their locked-down parents pin their artwork to lampposts on the high street. Little collectives of neighbours coordinate themselves on WhatsApp, collecting food and medicine for anyone in need. The elderly, the vulnerable, the man at number 41 with cancer – all now cocooned within their neighbours' arms, interlocked and steady to ensure that no one falls. When I ask my sister if I could borrow her rubber Crocs to wear inside the hospital, she immediately messages her street's Covid group and five pairs are delivered to her doorstep in under an hour, each now destined for staff in A&E.

Not once in my lifetime have I seen anything like this

grassroots eruption of improvised altruism. Communities coming together, the young and healthy offering to shop for those shielding, restaurants delivering mountains of takeaways to overworked hospital staff, everywhere the desire to be useful, to do something, to make it better, to help out. It startles and thrills me. There *is*, it turns out, such a thing as society. We *do* have more in common than that which divides us. Despite the country's scars, so deep-rooted, over Brexit, when the situation demands it – when what we face is life or death – most people act bravely and selflessly and with boundless initiative to protect ourselves and our neighbours from harm. And, just for a moment, it really does not seem to matter how we vote or what we do for a living. We are facing this adversity, by and large, as one. And there is a paradox with social distancing so unexpected, so hopeful, it makes me want to laugh out loud: we have never been closer while standing further apart.

When I happen to pull into our drive at eight o'clock in the evening of the last Thursday in March, I'm bewildered to find Dave, Finn and Abbey lining up on the doorstep. The idea of an impromptu ovation to express thanks to key workers has largely passed me by. A nice gesture, I may have thought, and lovely if it happened, but a gesture nonetheless, not anything of substance. But then, as I open the car door, applause begins to ripple and rise from my neighbours' doorsteps. Dave stares straight at me, grinning and clapping. Finn is belting his hockey stick against the wall. Abbey smashes a spoon on a saucepan with such fierce intensity she looks like a heavy metal drummer gone berserk in a pink nightie. My pre-school next-door neighbour appears actually delirious and though I know this is because it's a whole hour past his bedtime, his mad frenetic beating makes me choke up all the same. The entire village, it seems, is whooping and cheering, clanging and thumping, yelling 'N – H – S!' to the rooftops, and letting rip this most thunderous of thank yous to the nurses, the bus drivers, the cleaners, the porters, the shelf stackers, the doctors, the delivery drivers, the checkout staff, the police officers, the paramedics, the teachers, the carers and all of the other key workers who are out there amid the virus, braving Covid for the sake of others, playing their part to keep their neighbours safe and well.

And, honestly, I could fall to my knees at the sound. Its kindness and sweetness and community spirit overwhelm me with raw gratitude of my own. I stand on the tarmac, open-mouthed, tears streaming. All these people, this passion, this trenchant solidarity. It is the loveliest cacophony in the world.

'Have you noticed the people sitting in their cars in the car park?' I ask Mandi.

Her lips tighten for a moment and she slowly nods. 'It's so wrong, Rachel. Just wrong.'

It was eerie enough when hospital car parks transformed overnight from overcrowded rat traps, awash with queuing cars and irate drivers, into barren expanses of ghostland. With visitors banned, the cars stay away. Quickly, though, a new phenomenon emerged, perhaps the most plaintive sight I have ever seen in the hospital. A handful of parked cars began to appear each day, all of them angled so as to face the hospital. Their occupants sit impassively, sometimes for hours, staring at the threshold they are forbidden from crossing. The watchers hold vigil, strained and desperate, unable to resist being as near as possible to the person they love – a husband, a daughter, a sister, a father – now banished out of reach on a ward or in the ICU, often critically ill with Covid. They ache and ache for human contact – for holding, hugging, embracing, clinging on to – but the car park is as close as they can get. And so they sit in their vehicles, pulsing with longing, and suffer the absence of tactility.

During the Second World War, a young Scottish physician named Archie Cochrane was captured in Crete and became a medical officer in a string of prisoner of war camps, including some that were located in Nazi Germany. He went on to become a renowned epidemiologist, the father of modern evidence-based medicine. In the camps, though, the lessons he learned were not of numbers, but of the heart. In his autobiography, Cochrane describes caring for a moribund Russian prisoner, dumped by German soldiers on the ward late one night. Malnutrition was rife, medical supplies next to nothing. The patient shrieked in pain, yet Cochrane had minimal drugs to offer. With the ward full, and all the other patients sleeping, he put the young man in his own bedroom, diagnosing an aggressive pneumonia as the cause of his pain and screaming. What happened next was remarkable.

I had no morphia, just aspirin, which had no effect. I felt desperate. I knew very little Russian then and there was no one in the ward who did. I finally instinctively sat down on the bed and took him in my arms, and the screaming stopped almost at once. He died peacefully in my arms a few hours later. It was not the pleurisy that caused the screaming but the loneliness. It was a wonderful education about the care of the dying. I was ashamed of my misdiagnosis and kept the story secret.

For those hours during which he clasped a dying man in his arms, Cochrane administered that most vital of medicines – his human presence at his patient's bedside. It is a phenomenon we observe in the hospice time and again. In the end, as death bears down, there is almost no situation that cannot be made better by someone reaching out, with love and tenderness, towards one of our own. What we have, in our grief, is each other.

Yet Covid, as we have so painfully discovered, wrenches the dying away from those they cherish. We have been forced to exile the one group of people who matter more than anyone as death draws near. In this respect, our efforts to contain the virus are a violation of everything I know about good palliative care. And, like everything else with Covid, we are learning as we go, scrambling to catch up, amateurs whose expertise is being gleaned in real time, one patient after another. Nevertheless, we try. What else can we do but improvise, attempting to humanise the void imposed by necessarily draconian visiting restrictions and the physical barricades of PPE?

Mandi Kitching has intuited exactly how to set her collection of knitted hearts to work. Visiting may be curtailed, but the potency of symbols is not. When it becomes evident that a patient with Covid is beginning to die and Mandi meets their family, she offers them one of the little hearts. 'It's one of a pair,' she will say. 'We have another one here to leave in Dad's room. You can take this one away with you, and you'll know that he has the other and that it represents you, even though you can't stay for long in his room with him.'

Next, Mandi will place a little heart in the dying patient's room, perhaps on their pillow, their mattress or their bedside table. You could say this is nothing, perhaps even scoff at the gesture. A mere token, a cliché, an inch of knotted wool. But often, family members are deeply moved. Mandi has worked in palliative care long enough to know that the narratives we construct as our loved ones are being taken from us matter immeasurably. In this new hospital world of absence and barricades, the hearts speak of love, of kindness and compassion. They say that patients are still cared for as people.

When family members are unable to visit in person, Mandi will often show them the heart on a video call from inside the patient's room, and then, in another room many miles away, a man or woman may start to weep. I think about the smallness and slightness of these little scraps of wool that cannot ever make things right, yet possess undeniable power.

When I am scared and full of doubt – a daily occurrence of late – I find comfort in the opening verse of Emily Dickinson's hymn of praise to human hope:

> *'Hope' is the thing with feathers –*
> *That perches in the soul –*
> *And sings the tune without the words –*
> *And never stops – at all –*

Perhaps I am exhausted and sentimental from Covid, but Mandi's hearts, it seems to me, are an alternative metaphor for our capacity, despite everything, for hope. Across the country, there are thousands of deaths now, whole mountains of grief, and yet against them stand these scraps of wool, placed on pillows with the single aim of uniting the grief-stricken – tenuously, symbolically – with those they love and cannot bear to lose.

In the Covid ICU, a ventilator has been performing the work of breathing for Ken Wood for several days now. On day three of Ken's admission to intensive care, his daughter Laura takes a phone call from a doctor to explain that her father is deteriorating fast. As an ICU nurse herself, she knows what is coming. And sure enough come the words she dreads: 'Would you like to come in to see him? We're concerned he is not going to survive and we want to offer you and your mother that chance to be with him.'

Despite her shock, a part of Laura is lucid. She has been living with her mother, supporting her at home. She knows they both may well have been infected with Covid from her father and she cannot bear the prospect of putting others at risk. 'The last thing I wanted to do was bring it into the ICU,' she tells me. 'How could I live with myself if I did that?'

I have to take a breath at this admission of Laura's. She has just been told that her father may be dying. She has been offered a chance to see him one last time. But however much she yearns to be there at his side, she summons the strength to put the lives of others before her own. She declines a final chance to see her dying father in order to protect others, unknown, from a virus that could kill them.

Mercifully, the crisis passes. Ken's saturations begin to pick up. Though critically ill, he is no longer on the cusp of death. 'Be prepared for a long wait,' the ICU team tells Laura. 'He could be like this for weeks on the ventilator, even longer.'

In those weeks, someone calls Ken's home daily to update his family on his progress. Usually, Laura takes the calls, given her own expertise in intensive care. Such is Sanah Ali's eloquence that Laura assumes she must be an ICU outreach nurse, someone trained and experienced in communicating the worst. In fact, Sanah is a twenty-two-year-old medical student who nurtures a dream of specialising in disaster and conflict surgery, and who volunteered to help in any way she could, the moment Covid forced the medical school to close.

'I had no idea where I'd be useful,' she tells me. 'I felt uneasy but determined to be helpful. I was doing a placement in ED when things began to get serious. We'd walk past a room and see everyone being fitted with their PPE and we'd whisper to each other, "Oh God, this feels a bit dystopian."'

Sanah and four other students were assigned to the ICU relatives liaison team. The day after lockdown commenced, they arrived on the unit where a consultant psychiatrist, designated to mentor and support them, outlined how their role might work. 'We're not exactly certain yet, but we imagine you'll become very involved with the families of Covid patients in the ICU, updating them daily, potentially getting close to them.' She paused, as if noticing their age for the first time. 'Have you guys . . . dealt with much death?' There was silence for a second, then Sanah spoke up. 'You see it a little bit in the hospital, but I have no idea how I'm going to react, no. It's a bit scary.'

They say that learning medicine is a matter of 'see one, do one, teach one'. True to form, the five students were taken to the relatives liaison room where a team of ICU nurses were busy calling families. An ICU consultant happened to be holding a telephone conversation with a son about the fact that his father was so unwell it was time to consider withdrawing life support. 'She gave him so much time,' says Sanah. 'She was quiet and slow and thoughtful, every word mattered. It was my first experience of anything like that. Fifteen minutes later she called back to tell him his father had passed away. All of a sudden, the pandemic felt real. It was happening in Oxford. And I just wanted to do anything I could for these people, anything to alleviate their pain. I could see my role was important. We could do something that mattered, even if we couldn't change the outcome for the patients.'

Sanah and her colleagues observed a few more calls and quickly began making their own. 'We were certainly thrown in – but not quite in the deepest water. We were not expected to break the worst news.' Conversations rarely follow the rules though. Almost as soon as she started calling families, Sanah found herself being asked profound and awkward questions. 'I would have to talk about the fact that the person they loved was sick enough to die, that the next day or so was critical. I'd never done anything remotely like that before but there was no other option but to swim. If you don't do these calls then people are not going to know about their families. It's vital. It's someone's life. That responsibility kept me grounded. It's not about you, it's about them.'

Walking home one evening, Sanah felt numb. 'I realised I felt nothing at all. I couldn't go into the house. I sat on my doorstep for hours and then – it must have been 8 p.m. – I heard the sound starting up of the Thursday clap for carers. I thought of the people in the ICU I knew were going to die. I couldn't match it up. It was impossible.'

For Laura, Sanah's calls to update her on her father soon became a daily lifeline. 'She really knew us,' Laura says. 'She was our eyes and ears. She talked to me with such openness and kindness. I cannot believe a student was given that responsibility and built up a relationship with us with such incredible empathy.'

Across the NHS now – for all the husbands, wives, children and parents unable to say goodbye to those they love in person – a quiet revolution is underway. Using any means, we strive to bring humanity back to the spaces the virus has stripped bare. Our tools are uncertain and improvised. We are making it up as we go along. Phone calls, iPads, knitted hearts, recorded songs, laminated photos of our faces on our plastic gowns. We use whatever we can to draw people back together and we refuse to settle for despair.

9

Sacrifice

Courage. Kindness. Friendship. Character. These are the
qualities that define us as human beings, and propel us, on
occasion, to greatness.

R. J. PALACIO, *Wonder*

On the fourth floor of Manila's main hospital the heat is
oppressive, even at midnight. If you stepped outside into the
tropical night, sweat would bead your brow before you cleared
the ambulances. The 7000 or so small islands of the Philippine
archipelago are strung along the western arc of the Pacific
Ring of Fire, enduring typhoons, tsunamis, upheavals and
eruptions. People live under constant threat from molten rock
and tectonic shifts. Some 90 per cent of the world's earthquakes
and 75 per cent of its volcanoes occur along the Ring of Fire.
Cataclysm here is commonplace.

It's 1994. Ray Atienza-Hawkes is a newly qualified nurse,
halfway through a night shift. A young man in his early twenties, he can still hardly believe he is paid for doing a job he loves

with every fibre of his being. At first, the earthquake declares itself softly, imperceptibly. It builds, strengthens, a mug of tea starts to chatter and now the nurses flick glances of unease at each other. Is it happening? Yes, it's happening. The desks start to tremble. The patients cry out as the frames of their beds jangle. Dust drops from the ceiling. Tiles shatter as they fall. The lights die and the air fills with screaming. Stumbling through dust clouds, clutching walls to stay upright, Ray struggles through the debris towards his patients. The other nurses, he realises, have dived beneath desktops. It's not cowardice, it's good sense. In the Philippines, you are taught it as children. But Ray has acted on another, deeper impulse, an instinct that may be the death of him. He lurches on towards the beds, where drip stands crash and patients shriek into the darkness.

'I did it without thinking,' Ray tells me, smiling. 'I was an idiot, in a way. I know the other nurses thought I was. But how could I have left my patients? There was no way I could have done that.'

Some twenty-five years later, sacrifice is once more at the forefront of Ray's mind. He has proudly worked as a nurse for over two decades in Oxford University Hospitals NHS Foundation Trust. He is one of 18,000 Filipinos working in the NHS, third only to the numbers from Britain and India. We are lucky enough in Oxford to have over a hundred Filipino nurses and midwives in our hospitals.

When the pandemic began to kill NHS doctors and nurses, my colleagues and I were too stunned at first to think straight. 'Oh God,' we'd type on our phones to each other as another death was declared. They concussed you, these announcements, left you dumbstruck and stupefied. When the government responded with some oversized statistic about a trillion gloves or a gazillion aprons, I'd find myself stuck on the same incredulous loop. *But doctors and nurses are dying – right now – and their colleagues are begging for PPE they do not have.* Once, I had to pull over on the drive home from work. The news on the car radio stole even my expletives and, lost for words, I sat in a layby and wept for the latest nurses whose deaths had just been announced.

It took a little while for patterns to emerge. Perhaps we were too numb to see them. The staff who were dying came overwhelmingly from black, Asian and minority ethnic groups. No one understood precisely why, yet being white – with Covid as with so many things – appeared to confer a survival advantage. 'We all started asking, "What is happening? Why is this happening?"' Ray tells me. 'People were panicking. We were frightened but we carried on working. We couldn't just abandon the patients.'

Ray is the nurse manager of one of the most important parts of the John Radcliffe, the hospital's ambulatory assessment unit (AAU). In non-Covid times, unwell patients surge daily in high volumes through the unit for tests and assessments that cannot be carried out in their own homes. Often their problems can be diagnosed and solved in a day, without the patient ever having to face the risks and upheaval of a hospital admission. The unit performs an invaluable role in keeping people at home, close to those they love.

In Oxford, we are luckier than some. The AAU has all the protective kit it needs. No one here has ever had to resort to bin bags or homemade PPE. Nevertheless, Ray and his team are acutely aware that as their patients flow through the unit, any one of them could be harbouring the virus. 'You don't realise it at the time, but you are running on adrenalin and fear,' he says. 'Everyone knows someone affected by Covid. Even when you go home you can't shut down. The streets are empty. The deaths are on the news. You're surrounded by it wherever you go.'

Just before Easter, the whole world feels broken. Seventy-five thousand people have now died of Covid globally; 10,000 of those fatalities have occurred in Britain, a nightmarish number I can scarcely grasp. A world leader – our Prime Minister – has been rushed into intensive care and no one knows if he will ever re-emerge. Truly, in the words of Zadie Smith, a 'global humbling' is upon us.

And then, in Oxford, there is devastating news. 'It is with tremendous sadness that we announce the deaths of two members of staff, both of whom were porters at the John Radcliffe Hospital and both married to members of our nursing teams,' says the email sent out to every member of staff. The trust's CEO, Dr Bruno Holthof, goes on: 'We are a team and every single member of our team is precious.' And it is true. It was true before Covid and it is immeasurably truer now. Oscar King Junior and Elbert Rico were both Filipino men in their forties. Widely known and loved across the hospital, their deaths hurt every one of us.

Ray's community is shattered. The five Filipino nurses on his team are frightened. A member of Ray's own family dies from the virus and then a good friend and colleague is admitted to the Covid ICU. The threat that had once seemed so improbable, so distant, is now every bit as oppressive as the earthquakes in Manila all those years ago. And still Ray goes to work. 'I choose to be here, in a way, because it is the one normal thing

I have left. Coming here and doing my job is the one routine that hasn't been taken from me.'

One of the most loved members of the AAU team is sixty-two-year-old Philomina Cherian, an Indian nurse originally from Kerala. Initially, when she becomes unwell, lockdown has yet to even happen. She stays at home with her son and husband, hoping her symptoms will pass. But the act of breathing becomes ever more exhausting. When Philomina is finally admitted to the hospital in which she has worked for over a decade, Ray is worried sick. Quickly she is transferred to ICU. She spends the next fifteen days deeply sedated on a ventilator. Other members of staff have now been brought here too. The intensive care team are caring for colleagues whom they know and recognise and have worked with before.

On the AAU, Philomina is renowned for her warmth and kindness and everyone is willing her, please, to recover. One day the hospital's matron seeks out Ray in person. The briefest glance at her face and he knows it is no good. 'I'm so sorry,' she tells him. Ray gathers his team to break the unthinkable news. There is no sugar coating, no way to soften this blow. 'I've been told Philomina is unlikely to survive,' he says quietly. Her fellow nurses sit in silence and cry. 'You want to reach out to them, to hug them,' Ray tells me, 'and Covid means you can't. All you can do is hand out tissues. Everything that comes instinctively and naturally as a caring human being has been taken away by the pandemic.'

That night, Alice Warwick, the deputy sister in ICU, is leading the nursing team in the bay where Philomina lies. Once the decision has been made to withdraw her life support, the nurses know what is coming. 'There were no words,' Alice later says simply. 'Horrible, horrible, horrible.' With the utmost tenderness, each touch an act of love, they care for Philomina in the last hours of her life. And when, shortly after midnight, the agony is over, every member of the night shift who possibly can slips away from their role on the ICU to line the corridor through which she will shortly pass. Doctors, nurses, carers and porters stand in silence, faces rigid, heads bowed, to honour the courage and kindness and boundless heart of a woman who sacrificed her life to save others.

'In all my career as a nurse, this is the most difficult situation I've ever known,' Ray says. 'We lost one of our own, a nurse we loved, and I keep telling my team "It's OK not to be OK, it's OK to find it hard" but I don't think I've ever really asked myself if I am OK, genuinely OK. We're always being kind to other people, being nurturing, but to be able to do that we have to be kind to ourselves first. I don't think we're very good at that. We go back to work, we keep caring for patients. I'm trying to make sense out of what has happened and I can't. I can't process it. What will happen to the staff? Will everyone develop PTSD? Maybe we will all need therapy.'

Ray and I are talking in a room just big enough to contain a little sofa and two soft chairs. A low table lamp emits a warm glow. On the walls, the artwork is beautiful. In the wake of Philomina's death, the trust asked AAU staff what they needed, anything that might help. This space, came the answer, somewhere quiet and serene, a sanctuary to retreat to whenever the strains of the job demand it. Its creation, says Ray, has helped staff feel cared for. 'Most of all, though, we wanted to show Philomina's family how much she meant to us.' He shows me a remembrance book the staff have created for her family, each page a handwritten declaration of love and affection. 'I think making this collectively has helped us feel better. Small acts of kindness go a long way. Nurses know that better than anyone.'

He pauses. 'Why does it have to take a pandemic for people to be kind to each other?'

The UK is surpassing the apocalyptic death tolls we could not tear our eyes from in Italy. Nearly a thousand people in Britain are dying of Covid every day. The Prime Minister, mercifully, leaves intensive care but so many more patients remain. I don't know anyone who feels able to share what they see inside the hospital with their family back at home. I want to talk to Dave. I want to cry in his arms. But how could he understand, and why would I put him through that? On Easter Sunday, I receive a message from a friend in another trust who has been redeployed to work in their ICU. 'Please can I ask a huge favour?' it reads. 'I need a witness for signing my will. I'm trying to sort this out urgently at the moment. One of our colleagues just died in the ICU and a lot of us are sorting out legalities ASAP just in case.'

I call her back. Shreya is a mother with three children under ten. Her husband, like mine, has a non-medical job and I am guessing she may need to talk. Our stories tumble out, a torrent of words on both sides. The moment we start talking, it feels as though we'll never stop. 'It is absolute madness,' Shreya says. 'I mean . . . we have kids. What the hell are we doing, Rachel?'

We share our concerns that the public has not grasped how terrifying and arbitrary this illness can be. How young some patients are, how inexplicably they crash. We have never known such fear among our fellow doctors. None of us can say for certain that we will be spared.

175

One day I am chatting to one of the carers in the hospice. Tracey Allen has worked as a healthcare assistant in Katharine House for twenty-six years. She has the natural warmth and open features that inspire immediate trust – the kind of face a small child would instinctively run to, convinced they'd find a haven in her arms. We are talking about the moment when the nursing team were asked how they would feel about the hospice turning into a Covid response centre. 'I was absolutely terrified of getting it and taking it home to my family,' Tracey says. 'My daughter cried for two weeks when I told her. How can your child understand your desire to do something that could take you from them? But I said yes because this is what we do. I was proud to do it.'

If there is a diametric opposite to the technological wizardry of the ICU, it is embodied in Tracey. She provides intensive care of the human kind. 'I make a difference, I hope. I feel as though when patients come here, we put them back together again. They've been through so much and we try to give them the time and respect they need. I try to put myself in their shoes – how would I want that person to behave to me? You use touch, reassurance. We are the backbone. My role is to help people feel safe and cared for.'

She doesn't know it, but I try to emulate Tracey. I have watched the frowns and fretfulness of dying patients dissolve in real time as she instils the belief that she will be there for them, come what may. Now she is being torn by Covid in two different directions at once. 'As soon as someone with the virus coughs, your natural reaction is to run back. Normally my instinct is always to move in, to be closer, but with Covid it's to get further away. And that is horrible. The virus is a barrier between us and them.' Except, I have observed, even in these twisted times, Tracey and her team always seem to find a way to demonstrate their care.

One weekend, a young mother begins to deteriorate. Her daughters arrive with their father to say goodbye to Mummy, who is dying of both cancer and Covid. 'Those are beautiful dresses,' I say to the two little girls. One gazes up at me with the utmost solemnity. 'We're wearing our unicorn dresses to cheer up Mummy,' she tells me. But their matching purple-sequinned unicorns have to be hidden. I help the daughters one by one into flopping blue gloves and adult-sized protective aprons. Four sparkling ballet shoes peep out beneath swathes of NHS plastic. The girls' lips quiver when I help them into their masks. 'You are being so brave for your mummy,' I tell them.

If this feels hard, it is nothing compared to the difference the nursing team later makes. That night, the young woman becomes distressed. It is a wide-eyed anguish neither morphine nor midazolam touches. She implores the nurses to help her. There is no drug in the world that can anchor her here, staving off the moment she finally departs. And so the nurses come close, they lean in and cradle her. What they give in these moments is more potent than morphine. As for whether it violates a strict Covid code of infection control – well, maybe, but that depends on whether you believe this human closeness was necessary. To me, it is nothing less than an act of grace, a pinpoint of light in these dark times.

My journeys between work and home, these days, feel like interplanetary travel. The two worlds are light years apart. I no longer recognise, let alone feel at home in, the one my family inhabits. I find myself itching to get back to the hospital. Once inside, there is the instant relief of meaning, focus, purpose. The politicians and statistics and endless disputes recede and dissolve into thin air. Patients and colleagues are a living, breathing antidote to the shapeless anxiety that keeps me pacing the kitchen after dark. In the hospital, we think of nothing but the patient in front of us. We are granted the liberation of absorption. In here, at last, I can exhale.

Outside, Finn and Abbey revel in their own unexpected freedoms. Home schooling, for instance, is entirely compatible with spending whole days in pyjamas. Lunch, with careful tactics, can sometimes be composed exclusively of Pringles and marshmallows. Bedtimes are endlessly elastic. Dave's job, for now, is safe, though he is not entirely sure about being turned overnight into a 1950s housewife. ('You have total control of the kids, darling. Is that OK?' I asked, sounding sorry-not-sorry.) We have a little garden and, beyond that, the countryside. We are healthy, happy and can afford him being furloughed. We do not take lightly how privileged we are. 'So many people are going to lose their jobs, Rach,' Dave says one evening. The magnitude of pandemic losses, piling higher with each day that passes, is like nothing we have lived through before.

Sometimes I try to imagine the strangeness, for the wider public, of life under lockdown. Gruelling commutes and office gossip have been replaced by laptops, Zoom and discreet mugs of tea placed out of range of laptop cameras. There are no nights out, no sport, no movies, no browsing the shops, no live entertainment. Boredom and anxiety are rife. There is unexpected joy, for some, in densely concentrated family life. For others, this new intensity is dangerous and suffocating.

'Why has everyone gone mad for baking?' I ask Dave one day. The *New York Times* has picked up on our curious obsession with banana bread and sourdough in a piece they run with the headline 'Pandemic-Baking Britain Has an "Obscene" Need for Flour'. A traditional Oxfordshire flour mill is featured, with its owner, miller Emily Munsey, describing frantically hiring more staff and adding afternoon and night shifts to keep the mill running twenty-four hours a day, seven days a week, for the first time in its 125-year history. Dave gestures proudly to the kitchen cupboard where a kilogram of Wessex Mill flour sits smugly, like gold in a vault. He cycled 10 miles to a farm shop to buy it. It's Munsey who has given the *Times* its immortal headline. Despite the mill's best efforts, the British public is insatiable. 'Demand remains consistently obscene,' she tells the disbelieving *Times* reporter.

The real obscenity, one could argue, is that some of us are mourning our disrupted access to yeast while others are being laid off, taking their first trips to food banks, struggling with toddlers in high-rise bedsits, or being beaten up by their partners behind closed doors. We are in this together, the government tells us repeatedly, their mantra one of determined unity. But are we? Are the sacrifices really spread evenly?

The evening after the Prime Minister is discharged from intensive care, the BBC *Newsnight* presenter Emily Maitlis opens the programme with a blistering dissection of the recent rhetoric surrounding coronavirus. 'The language around Covid-19 has sometimes felt trite and misleading,' she states. 'You do not survive the illness through fortitude and strength of character, whatever the Prime Minister's colleagues will tell us. And the disease is not a great leveller, the consequences of which everyone – rich or poor – suffers the same. This is a myth which needs debunking. Those on the frontline right now – bus drivers and shelf stackers, nurses, care home workers, hospital staff and shopkeepers – are disproportionately the lower-paid members of our workforce. They are more likely to catch the disease because they are more exposed. Those in tower blocks and small flats will find the lockdown tougher. Those in manual labour won't be able to work from home.'

Maitlis's words do not merely strike a chord, they spread like wildfire. For although anyone clearly *can* succumb to this brutal disease – as the PM's fate has so unnervingly demonstrated – in no sense does this mean our chances of doing so are *equal*. Nor do we equally suffer the burdens and privations of the pandemic. Now that those workers once dismissed as 'low-skilled' have been rebranded as 'key workers', for example, they are rightly being lauded as essential lynchpins of British society. But will this new status result in commensurate pay rises, better terms and conditions of work, or even – most pressingly – in adequate PPE? For security guards, shelf stackers, cleaners and carers, viral loads of Covid are a daily reality. Some of us, statistically, are more likely to come out of this worse than others. Far from uniting the UK's deep-seated economic and social divisions, the pandemic is serving to exacerbate them. I notice the odd starry-eyed piece in the press about post-pandemic utopian futures, but I worry that history shows otherwise: that in times of momentous upheaval, power consolidates power.

However, with all the sacrifices we face, both collectively and as individuals, the overwhelming majority of Britons are behaving with striking decency, resolved for the moment to respect the constraints of lockdown in order to protect each other. Outside the hospital, with no awareness of its role, the whole city in one sense is caring for the patients on ventilators. It is thanks to people's willing and gracious retreat from the public sphere that NHS resources have not been overwhelmed. Without the emptied streets and deserted open spaces, it could be so hauntingly different. Invisible threads of everyday sacrifice tie the world outside to the one within the hospital. So many people are giving as they suffer.

It is nearly two weeks since Ken Wood arrived in the Covid ICU. In all that time, teams of doctors and nurses have sought to control every aspect of his physiology with obsessive attention to detail. This is how ICU saves lives. Tiny jobs, done well, repeatedly, the eye never leaving the ball. Ken's blood pressure, heart rate, urine output, blood biochemistry – all of it is being mathematically monitored, tracked, plotted and manipulated. The one thing – the only thing – beyond the intensivists' grasp is his brain, the body's most disobedient and ungovernable organ.

From the moment he was sedated and placed on a ventilator, Ken has inhabited a lurid world of visions, nightmares and hallucinatory horror. His brain is running amok. *Please God,* he prays in psychotic desperation. *Rescue me, please. I can't bear it.* He sees the ceiling above his bed physically rippling with anger and violence. The nurses are impostors, the ward a fake. He has been kidnapped and drugged by a gang of rogues intent on extortion. Helpless and immobilised inside a bogus hospital, he is doomed unless he pays an impossibly high ransom. Then there is a fairground in his room, clanking and shrieking. Lights flicker, voices screech, machines jangle. A presence looms over him, its voice hard and cruel. 'Who is going to save you now?' it sneers. In his delirium, Ken manages to reply: 'The God of Love whom I love and fear will save me.'

Day after day, Ken fails to improve. He lies in limbo in the hinterland dividing life from death by complex algorithms, elaborate engineering and a thousand daily acts of impeccable nursing care. The proning team gathers, six or eight of them in total. *On my count – one, two, three.* Expertly, gently, they manoeuvre Ken's frame on to its front, where he lies for sixteen hours before being manhandled back again.

For Ken's daughter, Laura, and his wife, Helen, each day is an agony of waiting. They try to keep their spirits up, they know they must stay strong. But it takes superhuman effort to resist catastrophising. Always, always, the televised death tolls. Those statistical abstractions of lives lost, families shattered. How are you meant to keep a level head when death writ large is paraded daily?

And then, one day, Ken begins to emerge from his nightmarish hallucinations. At first, he trusts no one. They may all be impostors, part of the criminal ring that has kidnapped him. Dazed, disorientated and deeply suspicious, he is barely able to slur words comprehensibly – and yet, despite everything, he lives. The ICU has kept him alive. Laura takes a call from Sanah Ali, the medical student who updates the Wood family daily.

'Sanah?' Laura says, breathless for news. 'How's he doing? What's the latest? Is he OK?'

There is the briefest of pauses, then the sweetest of words: 'I have some really good news, Laura. He's woken up.'

As Ken's lucidity improves, his thoughts turn to his wife. 'Where is Helen?' he asks. 'I want to talk to Helen.' Sanah, who is there to hear him utter those words, describes the moment to Laura. 'I saw true love today,' Sanah tells her, and through the receiver she hears Laura repeating the words to her mother. An eruption of sobs swiftly follows as both mother and daughter begin to take on board what has happened. Dad has woken up. Dad is going to live. *This is pure joy,* Sanah thinks to herself. *Whatever I go on to see and experience as a doctor, I will never, ever forget this moment.*

10

Human Factors

The pestilence is at once blight and revelation.

ALBERT CAMUS, *The Plague*

My husband, on occasion, can be inhuman. By this, I do not mean I married a barbarian, but that he possesses certain qualities so singular they mark him out, I'm convinced, as a human outlier. It's his experience of stress that's abnormal. In an excessively pressured situation – when stimuli crowd in, at high speed, from all sides – most people feel flustered and over-whelmed. The relationship between pressure and performance is defined by the eponymous Yerkes-Dodson law. In 1908, this pair of American psychologists hypothesised that our levels of performance increase with mental or physical arousal – but only up to a point. Once the levels of arousal become too high, we are too stressed to perform at our peak any longer, and our performance begins to decline. This happens to me regularly when trying to cook a roast dinner. As for attempting to drive through London, I'm doomed before I've even left the M25.

184

When placed under escalating pressure, Dave, however, finds that time seems to slow, not accelerate. He computes his options with an otherworldly calm. Indeed, ever since boyhood, Dave was drawn to one of the most stressful situations in which a human being can find itself. With single-minded zeal he pursued the goal of becoming an RAF fighter pilot. This entails flying jets at speeds considerably faster than the speed of sound, while wrenching yourself through the sky with such violence that your body must withstand centrifugal forces five or six times the pull of gravity. Most of us would lose consciousness long before we ever entered an aerial dog fight, let alone have the capacity to avoid crashing our Tornado F3 into the ground, or into another F3. A '2 v 2' – two pairs of fast jets in air combat against each other – can have combined speeds of 4000 miles per hour. I'll be frank. Even the *thought* of this makes me feel queasy. That my husband used to revel in such madness leads me to suspect that, genetically, he is ever so slightly mutant.

Even fighter pilots lose their composure, however. A few times every year, a split-second miscalculation during training costs one of them, somewhere in the world, their life. And even fighter pilots have to learn how to dog-fight. There was a time in his training when Dave attempted his very first proper aerial combat, a 2 v 2 in which the other jet in his team was being flown by his grizzled old-school flying instructor. 'I did not, it's fair to say, cover myself in glory,' Dave confessed when he told me this story. To his inexperienced eyes, the other three pilots possessed superhuman abilities to see. They could read the skies, second-guess the jets' locations, while Dave, hanging on for grim death, could barely function. 'I had no situational awareness at all. I hardly knew which way was up, let alone where to find my targets.'

In the post-mission debrief, Dave's instructor made his displeasure known in a scene most definitely worthy of *Top Gun*. In furious silence, bristling with rage, he stomped to the blackboard and drew a huge 'T' in white chalk. He then rubbed it out and drew a 'W'. This was erased and replaced by an 'A', and the 'A' in turn with a 'T'.

Finally, he turned to face my future husband. 'What are you?' he snarled.

'A twat, sir.'

'Yes, Flight Lieutenant. Yes, you fucking are. And if you ever fly like that again, you'll be chopped.'

And with that, the debrief was over.

In healthcare, just as in aviation, an inability to see the big picture can be fatal. An entire industry exists these days aimed at bringing aviation ergonomics – so-called 'human factors' – to bear upon the lethal consequences for patients of their clinicians becoming too overwhelmed with stress to function safely. An official NHS England report on human factors states that: 'delivering healthcare can place individuals, teams and organisations under pressure. Staff have to make difficult decisions in dynamic, often unpredictable circumstances. In such intense situations, decision making can be compromised, impacting on the quality of care, clinical outcomes, and potentially causing harm to the patient ... By acknowledging human limitations, Human Factors offers ways to minimise and mitigate human frailties, so reducing medical error and its consequences.'

Every doctor, at some stage in their career, has felt the sickening sensation of being blinded at work by sensory, physical or emotional overload. An essential challenge for any safety critical industry – medicine as much as aviation – is to ensure that no individual faces systemic pressures of such severity that their performance may be dangerously compromised. Even at the best of times, NHS understaffing can make this a tall order. If a pilot calls in sick one day, his co-pilot is not expected to fly the aeroplane single-handed. But in the NHS, there is no equivalent of an aeroplane being grounded. All too frequently in a system short of tens of thousands of frontline staff, one doctor or nurse is forced to take on the workload of two, with all the additional stresses that entails.

By early April, as cases of coronavirus skyrocket, it is already becoming painfully apparent that the NHS as a whole may be facing its own grim version of an aerial dog fight. Hospital managers and senior clinicians are rightly racing to clear space for the incoming waves of infected patients. Their overwhelming priority is ensuring that oxygen, ventilators and ICU beds will not run out. But though this single-minded focus is crucial for those who could die without intensive care, it neglects other patients, unseen and unheard. Just like my rookie husband in his first air-to-air combat, the pandemic is costing the NHS and the government their peripheral vision.

Suddenly, the press is full of shocking headlines such as 'Elderly Abandoned to Worst the Virus Can Do', 'Sacrificing the Elderly' and 'A Callous Betrayal of Our Most Vulnerable'. They refer to the spectacle of first hundreds, then thousands of care home residents dying as Covid tears through their homes despite the best efforts of staff. The details are painful to read. Hospital Covid tests are taking five days or more to be processed by a tiny number of centralised labs. Hospitals are therefore being driven to discharge patients back into care homes without knowing for sure that the patients are free from Covid.

The government has already insisted this does not matter. There was no need to test care home residents prior to discharge from the hospital, they told us, because even those who were infected could 'be safely cared for in a care home'. But this could not have been more wrong. Care homes have not been provided with remotely adequate supplies of PPE. Helpless staff are using bin bags, washing-up gloves and even sanitary towels as makeshift masks to try to avoid spreading infection among the residents for whom they care. Those residents – the very old, the very sick and people with disabilities – are precisely the population most at risk of dying from Covid. Yet far from being cocooned, as the government promised they would be, they are being incarcerated with Covid.

On 22 April, the manager of a care home in Ealing agrees to speak anonymously to the *Guardian* newspaper. Her words encapsulate the unfolding national horror: 'I have never written so many death notifications in such a short time. Every member of staff is lost. They don't know what to do. In one of our units with twenty-one residents, we lost nine people in three days. It's OK when you hear the numbers on TV. They are removed from reality. One day a resident was walking around with a mild temperature. I went home and the next morning they were dead . . . The care home sector needs help: staff, protection and volunteers. This has been going on since the beginning of April and I still think we are heading for the worst.' In predictable style, the written response from the Department of Health and Social Care includes a very large yet irrelevant number. 'So far we have delivered nearly 1 billion items of PPE across the health and social care system within England,' its author writes as if hoping, perhaps, for a round of applause.

A few weeks later, when giving testimony to the House of Commons Science and Technology Committee in early June, Professor Neil Ferguson, the epidemiologist whose calculations finally led to lockdown, will make waves when he explains that if the government had imposed lockdown one week earlier 'we would have reduced the final death toll by at least a half'. That week's delay could have cost up to 20,000 lives, the calculation based on the well-recognised fact, at the time, that the outbreak was doubling in size every two to three days. 'So whilst I think the measures, given what we knew about this virus then, in terms of its transmission, were warranted,' Ferguson will explain, 'certainly had we introduced them earlier, we would have seen many fewer deaths.'

Less widely reported, but no less shocking, will be his comments on the deaths of care home residents. 'We made the rather optimistic assumption that somehow the elderly would be shielded,' Ferguson will tell MPs, adding that this 'simply failed to happen'. Although the government's Scientific Advisory Group for Emergencies (SAGE) had 'anticipated in theory' the risk to people living in care homes and discussed this in meetings as early as February, no definitive action was taken. The 'only way you can really protect care homes is to do extensive testing to make sure it doesn't get in', Ferguson will conclude. Yet this is testing that never happens.

All this is to come, but in late April none of it is being admitted openly. I feel as though I am somehow complicit in a full-scale betrayal of the country's most vulnerable citizens.

Care home residents are being thrown to the wolves. It is not that I believe hospitals necessarily could have done any differently – not with the crippling inertia of centrally imposed five-day testing turnarounds – but that we *all*, myself included, should have raised the alarm sooner. Every one of us, from the Prime Minister down, should have noticed what was happening and, better still, predicted and planned for it. The country has *not* protected its least visible members, who are dying in care homes in appalling numbers. And this is not a party political point. Over the past two decades – half that time under Conservative governments, half under Labour – there have been seventeen white papers, green papers and state reviews of social care funding. What unites *both* parties during this time is prevarication and a failure to take decisive political action to make Britain's broken care system fit for purpose. Instead it limps on, fragmented and neglected, hollowed out by austerity, underfunded to the point of collapse. Meanwhile, governments from across the political spectrum keep avowing with fanfare to fix this scandal once and for all – and keep breaking those promises with impunity.

When Susan Price, at the age of fifty-three, received the news that her breast cancer had recurred, she reacted with characteristic defiance. 'Right. Come on then, let's get the bastard,' she said to her oncologist in late 2019. I am phenomenally healthy, she told herself. I walk, I run, I go to the gym. If this cancer is in my bones, then we need to hit it with everything we can.

Chemotherapy was duly planned for the start of February 2020. Susan resolved to enjoy the best Christmas imaginable with her husband and three grown-up children before subjecting herself once more to the rigours of treatment. 'At least that was the plan,' she tells me wryly. 'But then, very softly to begin with, Covid began rearing its head.'

As her vague awareness of a virus in China turned into animated discussions with her oncologist about the pros and cons of reducing the usual doses of her imminent chemotherapy regime, Susan began to feel daunted. 'The stories from Italy were horrendous. There was talk in the media of the NHS collapsing. I agreed to the dose reduction, fully aware this meant I wouldn't be hitting my cancer with all I should, because I was absolutely terrified of catching Covid with a compromised immune system.'

Susan intuited precisely where she stood in the pandemic's patient hierarchy. 'Here I was, a middle-aged woman dying from metastatic cancer. I wasn't the cute child or the vibrant twenty-year-old who would have everything thrown at them. I was very low down the list. I was the lowest priority.'

As I listen to Susan, I find myself wincing. No doctor wants to be part of a system which does its utmost for some patients, yet casts others aside. But Covid has overturned everything. Whether consciously or not, utilitarian as well as clinical assumptions are being made about how to minimise overall harm. Susan herself accepted this early on. 'I understood that this was a real time of crisis,' she tells me. 'You triage, you have to make decisions. Some level of prioritisation is necessary, and if I were a doctor, I would have done the same. Therefore, it was incumbent upon me to do what I could to protect myself. I wasn't self-pitying, I was realistic. You are way down this list, and you are going to have to do what you can to protect yourself.'

Weeks before the government imposes lockdown, Susan retreats reluctantly inside her home, emerging only for her doses of chemotherapy. She cannot understand the lack of urgency and leadership on social distancing. 'We are a decent, compliant people. We like to do the right thing and we want to be good. All we needed was someone telling us what to do, telling us why we needed to do it and being honest with us. We'd have done whatever was asked of us if we'd thought it would help save lives. I kept thinking, Why isn't the government taking control?'

Pain begins to flicker and flare in Susan's chest and abdomen. A scan reveals that, despite her chemotherapy, the cancer is continuing to spread. Her liver and lungs are now affected. Then, despite her best efforts at shielding, she develops a persistent cough and has difficulty breathing. Increasingly, she finds herself fighting for air. Terrified that she has caught Covid, she dials 999. For a moment, when they arrive in full PPE, the paramedics appear on the brink of taking her to hospital. Then she mentions she is on palliative chemotherapy for metastatic cancer. Suddenly, everything changes. 'In normal circumstances, we'd take you in,' the paramedics tell her. 'But there's Covid in there. It would be much better for someone like you to stay at home.'

Someone like you. On one level, Susan recognises that these comments are well intentioned, aimed no doubt at protecting her from infection with Covid. At the same time, she fears that the paramedics have become mid-pandemic hospital gatekeepers. 'I believed I was effectively being told not to waste NHS resources. I felt as though someone had opened a bin and just chucked me in it.'

Susan remains at home where she struggles on with pain, nausea and breathlessness. Further conversations with her oncologist lead her to make the sombre decision to abandon chemotherapy, which is doing little to arrest the growth of her tumours while causing ever more debilitating symptoms. Now there is nothing standing between Susan and dying. Her cancer is running its course, unimpeded. Cut off at home in isolation with her family, she starts to feel overwhelmed with pain and fear. 'I was terrified. I was losing my dignity. I started begging my family to call Dignitas. I would have taken my life right then if I could have done.'

Eventually, Susan's family call the paramedics again and this time she is admitted to hospital. In her distraught, dehydrated and desperate state, it feels, she says, 'like being dropped into Hades'. Blood leaks from the numerous puncture marks on her arms where a doctor has attempted and failed to cannulate her. Anonymous staff in PPE rush past. Screams and moans split the air. This is where I'm going to die, she thinks to herself, listening to people howling, staring at doctors in masks, with blood all over my hands.

When I meet Susan for the first time, it is several days after her transfer from the hospital to the hospice. She still appears wan and haunted by fear, but both her mood and symptoms have begun to improve. A turning point, it seems, was the morning after she arrived in hospital. A nurse named Mel appeared at her bedside. Susan laughs as if faintly embarrassed by the way the superlatives gush from her mouth. 'It was like an angel had just walked in,' she tells me. 'It felt like I'd just met a human being for the first time. She just stopped and looked at me properly. She looked into my eyes and she saw *me*.'

Susan immediately noticed that Mel elected not to tower over her, but rather sat down on a chair where she waited and patiently listened. 'I wanted someone to scoop me up. It really doesn't matter if you are three or fifty-three, it's still the same feeling. She saw how scared I was and she scooped me up and somehow gave me hope and confidence. I was still dying, of course, but now I had faith that someone wanted to help me.'

In the hospice, this attentiveness continues. Through tiny acts of thoughtfulness – fresh jugs of iced water, little servings of ice cream – the staff are managing to repair her shattered trust. I find it hard to hear Susan's reflections on how Covid has transformed her experience of healthcare. 'The virus has probably shortened my life by making full-dose chemotherapy too risky. It has certainly damaged my mental health, creating unimaginable stresses by physically taking away my support networks. It has stolen part of my life and impacted hugely on my experience of death. It left me totally alone and cut off from professional support when I had never needed it more. Covid made things unbearable. I love my life – but not at all costs. You think the NHS will always be there for you. You think it is this whole incredible edifice, but then coronavirus comes along and it all falls apart like dust.'

A part of me longs not to share those words here. I am so intensely proud of everything that NHS and care staff *have* managed, at such risk to themselves, to achieve for their patients. Highlighting any mid-pandemic shortcomings feels almost like an act of betrayal. But when I look in Susan's eyes, at their intelligence and clarity, I know I do not have a choice. She has, at most, a few weeks to live. Yet she is adamant about wishing to share her story. She has chosen to devote a portion of the precious time she has left to recounting her experiences in the hope that others may learn from them. At the very least, we owe it to her to listen. For me to censor her words would be unthinkable.

The painful truth in late April is this. The NHS, by the skin of our teeth, has not been overwhelmed by patients with Covid – but only because we have suspended much of our 'normal' activity while cobbling together several thousand extra ICU beds. Patients with cancer, care home residents – anyone, in fact, not critically ill with the virus – is at risk of slipping through the cracks in our remaining services. None of us intended to abandon anyone. Staff are working as hard as they have ever done in their lives. Yet abandoned is precisely how patients like Susan feel. There will be so much to learn from these weeks of crisis, so much in the future we could do differently and better. An essential first step is listening to the experiences of patients and loved ones who felt cut adrift mid-pandemic.

On the last day of April, a shimmering alloy of sunshine and showers, the Prime Minister is sufficiently recovered from his own hospitalisation with Covid to chair that day's pandemic press conference. Flanked by his chief scientific and medical advisers Patrick Vallance and Chris Whitty, Boris Johnson's oratory is rousing. 'We have so far succeeded in the first and most important task we set ourselves as a nation,' he declaims, 'to avoid the tragedy that engulfed other parts of the world.' This success has been demonstrated, he continues, by three key facts: 'At no stage has our NHS been overwhelmed. No patient went without a ventilator. No patient was deprived of intensive care.'

The language shocks me. The reality is that the UK now has the world's third-highest death toll from Covid and is on course to be the worst-hit country in Europe. Our 66 million inhabitants make up less than 1 per cent of the world's population, yet we have had to date more than 10 per cent of the recorded deaths from coronavirus worldwide. And today's UK mortality statistics were published before the Prime Minister's press conference. He would therefore have known that, as of 30 April, a total of 26,614 people in Britain had died of Covid. That's 26,614 families that are bereaved and grieving. It is an extraordinary context in which to speak of 'success'. How very cheap, how spectacularly expendable, one human life must be, I think, if the avoidance of tragedy is consistent with the deaths of nearly 27,000 people.

That night, I keep thinking of the patients I have cared for in the preceding weeks, all of them lacking the physiological reserves to withstand mechanical ventilation. It is not that they were denied intensive care due to rationing, but that the treatment was likely to cause more harm than good. Yet this should never have meant that their lives mattered less. I realise, perhaps belatedly, that all this dying on the margins, far away from any ICU, was overlooked from the outset. The first government slogan said it all. *Stay at Home. Protect the NHS. Save Lives.* We were being urged to protect an inanimate system, not people. The country has been throwing its all at building structural capacity so that those young and healthy enough to benefit from intensive care can receive it. A good aim, an admirable aim – except for all those it excludes. The elderly, the disabled, the frail and infirm, this second tier of lower-priority citizens. Where were *they* in the pandemic planning? Who, as the Prime Minister might put it, was considering the rest of the herd?

*

The revelations are too fast, too furious. Everything we learn comes at us in a rush, a supersonic inundation of data. If we were at the top of our game, it might feel different, but so many staff are already stunned and reeling, myself most definitely included. In a pandemic, just getting through the day can be an ordeal, let alone keeping your balance as you discover, for the umpteenth time, that what you thought you knew has just been upended. Days and nights are bleeding into each other and still the patients keep coming. There is no end in sight. 'I have to hide inside now if I'm at home on a Thursday evening,' one colleague tells me. 'I don't deserve to be clapped by the public. I'm knackered and I just wish it would end. I'm not a hero at all.'

Though gruelling, this concertinaed learning is vital. Medicine, as with any science, is inherently iterative. As new data emerge, what was once gold-standard medical practice can swiftly be rendered obsolete. And this is precisely how stand-ards improve for patients. Being open about our mistakes and shortcomings is crucial for doing better next time. Refining our practice depends on it.

As the end of April approaches, we remain deeply immersed in the pandemic. I cannot claim distance or objectivity, let alone any wisdom. Most days, I wish it would all go away and that I could simply hug my mum and friends again. But if there is one word that encapsulates for me the preceding month of accelerated dying, it is 'awful', in the original sense. The past four weeks have inspired fear, wonder, trepidation, dread, and a kind of grimly reverential respect. I am full of awe. I am awestruck. Dying is dominating the national conscious-ness like never before in my lifetime. As a country, we have been forced – however reluctantly, however unwillingly – to confront our own mortality. Perhaps then, when one day the pandemic passes, we will emerge transformed for the wiser.

Not so long ago, death was an intimate business. As a small child, for example, my grandmother woke up one morning to find her sister had died in the bed beside her. In Victorian England, this was by no means unusual. Typically, we left the world as we entered it, wrapped not in hospital sheets but in the warmth and intimacy of our own homes. Birth and death were witnessed experiences. We observed dying up close, we knew what it looked like. We smelt and heard and touched it. And then, as modern medicine became increasingly institutionalised, we lost that familiarity with the process of dying. Professionals intervened – paid doctors and nurses. Death, in essence, was outsourced to others. In the late twentieth century it became possible to live your entire life without ever directly setting eyes on death, despite half a million people dying in Britain annually. Death evolved from a natural and domestic occurrence into something fearful and foreign from which many of us now recoil. Even some doctors have a habit of tip-toeing away from the daunting business of their patients' dying.

Coronavirus has overturned all this. Now, once again, whether we like it or not, death is all around us. Although physically the dying takes place behind closed doors, nearly everyone knows someone who has lost a loved one to Covid. Death dominates the headlines, fires up social media. Television news is wall-to-wall Covid. You are mortal, the world screams in our faces. Pretend otherwise all you like, but one day you too will die.

The renewed public focus on dying may prove to be one

of the positives to come from the awfulness. Compassion in Dying, for example, an organisation which campaigns to encourage people to consider and document their end-of-life wishes, reports a 160 per cent rise in the number of living wills completed via its website between 20 March and 20 April, compared with the same period last year. Otherwise known as 'advance directives', these documents allow people pre-emptively to refuse life-prolonging treatments, such as CPR, should they become unable to make or communicate their wishes in the future. The organisation also reports a 226 per cent increase in people completing 'advance care plans', which, though not legally binding, allow people to record anything that matters to them about their future care, such as where they would like this to be, who they would like to be present and even what brings them the greatest joy – be it fresh air, nature or jazz on the radio. Increased advance care planning gives patients a sense of control and agency, and enables better communication between doctors, patients and families. The alternative, too often, is the rushed and panicked conversations when someone, suddenly, becomes gravely ill and their family discover with a sickening lurch that they have no idea about their wishes.

The most important learning to come from the pandemic will arise, perhaps, from its greatest cruelty, the unspeakable pain for so many families of being unable to be present when their loved one dies, or to mourn together with others after-wards. So often, I find I am updating anxious spouses, sons or daughters by telephone who are themselves self-isolating. They have no one to hug, no warm human presence to cling on to. Should any of them be permitted into hospital to visit their loved one with Covid, they will be told that they must now self-isolate at home for at least fourteen days. Thus, the newly bereaved are driven behind closed doors where they must suffer alone, stripped of the rituals and basic comforts of grieving such as congregating with others, swapping stories about the life of the one who has been lost, honouring them with shared memories and affection.

Kathryn de Prudhoe is a psychotherapist in Leeds whose parents divided their time between living in France and in a holiday caravan close to their daughter and grandchildren. In March, as concerns around coronavirus escalated, her parents flew back to the UK. 'I thought we would all be safer if we were all near each other in the UK,' Kathryn tells me. 'It never crossed my mind that my parents could end up at risk from getting on that plane or being in an airport.'

A few days after he arrived back in Leeds, Kathryn's father, Tony, began to feel unwell. Kathryn assumed that even if he did have Covid, being a fit and healthy sixty-year-old he would soon shrug it off. With lockdown imposed, she relied on telephone updates from her mother to check how he was faring. Although sufficiently unwell to be bedbound, Tony followed the advice he was given to stay at home, take paracetamol and drink plenty of fluids. 'One day, though, when I spoke to Mum, she started crying. She was so worried about Dad. This wasn't normal. When I look back I wonder why I didn't do something. Why didn't I call an ambulance? Or go inside the caravan to see him? I think I just obeyed the rules without thinking. I think we all followed the rules because we wanted to do the right thing.'

Thirty-six hours later, Kathryn's husband broke the devastating news that Tony had been rushed into hospital overnight.

When he collapsed in the bathroom, Kathryn's mother had had no option but to call the paramedics. In hospital, Tony was found to have severe Covid and was moved to the ICU. He had also suffered a stroke and a heart attack. For the next three days, as Tony continued to deteriorate, Kathryn would visit her mother, but never ventured inside her caravan. Dutifully, they would sit outside in garden chairs positioned three metres apart, hoping and yearning for good news from the hospital. But Tony was placed on a ventilator and given a 20 per cent chance of survival. The family were advised to prepare for the worst. 'Even when they told us they were going to withdraw Dad's life support, no one from the hospital offered us the chance to come in,' says Kathryn. 'No one suggested a video call or a phone call. And we just meekly complied. We thought it was what we had to do. We were obedient and I never even thought to question it.'

Once they had been told by telephone that Tony had been disconnected from his ventilator, the two women sat in the open air and waited. 'I kept thinking of the last three days when he'd been totally alone, surrounded by strangers. His lungs were filled with fluid, he'd had a bleed on the brain. It must have been physical torture and then, at some point, on top of all that, he would have known he was dying. I cannot bear to think of him there all alone.'

When, forty minutes after the first, the second call came to tell them Tony had died, Kathryn's and her mother's sobs could be heard across the caravan park. 'We were sitting outside for all the world to see. We had no privacy, we couldn't hug, we were out there on display.' For the next eleven days, fourteen days from the date of Tony's positive Covid test, his wife remained isolated inside the caravan. Kathryn would visit once a day to sit with her outside, but otherwise she was entirely alone, grieving in the absolute absence of others.

'When her self-isolation ended, I could see she was traumatised. She was like a small child wanting to be held and comforted. Her crying was desperate. Grief is messy at the best of times, but Covid bereavement is exceptionally complex. We were denied every ritual. We hadn't said goodbye, we hadn't prepared, we didn't see Dad's body, we didn't prepare the body, we weren't even allowed to go to the crematorium, not a single one of us. The funeral parlour allowed us in briefly for a twenty-minute service and I gave my dad a eulogy, but this was nothing like the celebration of the life of a man who was loved, the honouring of a person that a funeral should be. It has been and remains unbearable.'

Before this virus swept the world, medicine managed the process of dying with varying degrees of sensitivity. Although, at its best, a hospital environment *can* permit tenderness and intimacy at the end of life, too often these qualities are absent. A hospital death is often a rushed, chaotic, machine-dominated affair with little space or time for personal touches. The deathbed estrangements enforced by Covid have taken impersonality to an extreme and unprecedented degree. The pandemic has been a crash course in how to create the most traumatic conditions for bereavement imaginable. If, as clinicians, we are to take anything from its devastating impact on families, it is surely that we need to do all we can in future to bring the dying and their loved ones closer together.

In 2018, an American fan of the great singer-songwriter Nick Cave reached out to him via his website. Like Cave, Cynthia from Shelburne Falls, Vermont, had suffered several deeply painful bereavements. Cave himself had lost his young son, Arthur, in profoundly traumatic circumstances when he fell to his death from a cliff aged only fifteen. The reply Cave sent to Cynthia was so heartfelt and open and strikingly beautiful, it was instantly shared around the world. 'There is a vastness to grief that overwhelms our minuscule selves,' Cave wrote. 'We are tiny, trembling clusters of atoms subsumed within grief's awesome presence.'

I think of Cave's words often these days. He had been asked by Cynthia whether he ever sensed the spiritual presence of his son. His answer speaks to all we have lost in these bewildering and disturbing times, to everything we collectively grieve for. Normality. Familiarity. Financial and psychological security. The freedom to step outdoors when you want to. A world no longer coated in microbial poison. A daily routine. A trip to the movies. The indecent pleasure of office gossip. The confident purchase of toilet paper.

My daughter Abbey is asked to write a poem about lockdown for her English homework. She is missing, I discover, her friends and school pasta:

> We are racing around, squealing like pigs,
> Feet stamping the ground and snapping twigs.
> Now we laugh and have a munch:
> We love our delicious school lunch.
> I am tucked up cosy in my bed,
> Dreaming of what I could do instead,
> And I stare at the silver moon above
> And think of all the things I love.

I am temporarily floored by my daughter's expression of yearning. Losses stack up all around me. Some days it is easy to feel overwhelmed and hopeless – and this is even without personal bereavement. For those, like Kathryn de Prudhoe, whose loved ones have died of this terrible disease, in terrible isolation, the pain is scarcely imaginable. It takes Nick Cave, elaborating on the death of his son, to give me sense and perspective. His letter to Cynthia goes on: 'Dread grief trails bright phantoms in its wake. These spirits are ideas, essentially. They are our stunned imaginations reawakening after the calamity. Like ideas, these spirits speak of possibility . . . It is their impossible and ghostly hands that draw us back to the world from which we were jettisoned; better now and unimaginably changed.'

Now, on this last day of April 2020, there are over 26,000 families in Britain like Kathryn's, crushed and crumpled beneath grief's awesome power. They are lonely, scarred, aching and bleeding. The soothing rituals of loss have been replaced with emptiness and trauma. And yet, just weeks into our hellish immersion, everywhere, already, and with astonishing agility, people are doing their utmost to make things better. From the notices on lampposts asking neighbours if they need assistance to the tiny crocheted hearts connecting dying patients to their families. From the gorgeous, uplifting, weekly claps for key workers to the donated iPads that connect the hospital to the world outside its walls. From the Easter eggs and doughnuts dropped off for famished hospital staff to Captain Tom and the millions of pounds he is raising by walking laps of his garden. From the free fast-food coffees and NHS supermarket hours to the children making visors in their local Scout huts. All of these tiny eruptions of kindness. We are learning and striving, with imagination and empathy, to help each other, together.

Whatever else we may learn from this pandemic, here is what I know now. That in the preceding month I have seen purer and more concentrated human decency than I ever dared to believe was possible. That this worst of times has brought forth our best. And that people, fundamentally, are good.

Epilogue

Anyone with gumption
and a sharp mind will take the measure
of two things: what's said and what's done.

SEAMUS HEANEY, *Beowulf*

It is August 2020. Britain is fractious, frustrated and sizzling with enmity. Masks, an uncontentious matter when worn by clinicians, have become a flashpoint in a new cultural war. From the moment the government insisted we wear face coverings to protect others in shops and on public transport, they have been decried by a furious libertarian tendency as tools of a lily-livered nanny state intent on violating our most basic freedoms. The blistering heatwave does not help. We simmer and wilt with sweaty scraps of cloth across our mouths and noses doing nothing for anyone's temper.

The lockdown is all but over. We can eat out, drink out, go to cinemas and gyms again, and schools are on the brink of reopening. For weeks we haven't seen a single new patient in the hospital with Covid. The daily death tolls are now in single figures. We know though, from the Office for National

Statistics, that the total number of excess deaths in the UK during the pandemic, whether from Covid or other causes, stands at 65,000. England has the worst excess death toll of any country in Europe. More people have died of the virus than lost their lives during the whole of the Blitz. Rates of mental illness have soared, the economy has tanked, and over 600 health and care workers have died, some of whom openly begged for proper PPE before Covid cost them their lives. There is, it is fair to say, much to feel angry about.

An invisible speck of not-quite-life has caused whole human societies to grind to a halt. As of August 2020, deaths may be down, but cases are rising. We have no idea what lies ahead this winter. Nearly six months into the pandemic, the 'world-beating' Covid test-and-trace infrastructure the government loudly promised is yet to materialise. Worse, the precarious nature of PPE supplies has not remotely gone away. Each week, hospices like mine request the stock they need. Sometimes, if you are lucky, you get what you order – those 2000 sets of gloves required to function safely, for example. At other times there are no gloves at all. Occasionally, 4000 pairs may randomly arrive. There is no national procurement system, no proper supply chain, no robust and sustainable system for delivering PPE at all. How can this be? I think over and over. Has the government learned nothing, even now, about infection control?

Globally, the delusion that we are in control of our destinies has been exposed as such in blistering detail. All our certainties, our hubris, have come tumbling down. In our impotence, the instincts to blame and lash out are powerful. There is an equal hunger to make sense of the devastation unleashed by the virus. Sometimes I think the whole country is grieving.

Epilogue

Calls from bereaved families grow ever louder for an urgent public inquiry into what went wrong, and why, but the Prime Minister is yet to meet with them. When asked by journalists if he is ashamed of England having the highest number of excess deaths in Europe, Boris Johnson doubles down on his positive spin, boasting of the country's 'massive success' in bringing numbers down.

Despite all the talk of being 'in it together', it has become abundantly clear that the burden of illness and death due to Covid is not being shouldered equally. Evidence shows that if you live in socioeconomically deprived areas, come from black, Asian or minority ethnic (BAME) communities, or work in professions like social care, you are, quite simply, at greater risk. People from BAME backgrounds, for example, are around twice as likely to die from Covid than people who are white. It is unclear what measures, precisely, the government has instituted to try and minimise these racial disparities.

Kathryn de Prudhoe, still shell-shocked by grief, has joined 1800 other families to form the campaign group Covid-19 Bereaved Families for Justice UK. Her motivation – the 'last straw', as she told me – was the revelation in late May that the Prime Minister's chief adviser, Dominic Cummings, broke lockdown rules to travel 260 miles from London to Durham while infected with Covid, then took his family on a day out to a beauty spot during his recuperation. The news was met with an outpouring of anger from ordinary people who *had* conscientiously followed the rules. People not permitted to be there when their parents, children or partners died; or to attend funerals; or to visit elderly parents in care homes; or to greet newborn babies; or to be present at births.

When Johnson defiantly stood by his man, insisting that Cummings had behaved 'responsibly, legally and with integrity', Kathryn was compelled to vent her feelings in an article for the *Huffington Post*: 'The Prime Minister's suggestion that Cummings did what any caring father would do only adds insult to injury. My family and I followed the rules to the letter, even in the most horrific circumstances. We did what was needed to safeguard the wider community believing it was the right thing to do . . . Cummings has behaved with complete disrespect for our loss and sacrifice, and completely undermined the public health message to stay at home during this pandemic. The Prime Minister, and the government ministers defending him, are undermining the efforts of millions of people who, like me, have spent months in lockdown making their own sacrifices.'

The collective incredulity of doctors and scientists was summed up when Stephen Reicher, Professor of Social Psychology at the University of St Andrews and a member of the SAGE subcommittee advising the government on behavioural science, tweeted his response to watching the Prime Minister defending Cummings on live television. 'In a few short minutes tonight, Boris Johnson has trashed all the advice we have given on how to build trust and secure adherence to the measures necessary to control Covid-19. Be open and honest, we said. Trashed. Respect the public, we said. Trashed. Ensure equity, so everyone is treated the same, we said. Trashed. Be consistent, we said. Trashed. Make clear "we are all in it together". Trashed.' He concluded, with devastating understatement, 'It is very hard to provide scientific advice to a government which doesn't want to listen to science.'

Epilogue

Stoking Reicher's anger was his expert understanding of the centrality of trust to surviving a pandemic. What moral authority does a government retain to impose rules upon the general population when its most powerful adviser has transparently broken them, yet been backed to the hilt by his boss? Why, in short, would anyone continue to trust and obey a Prime Minister perceived to have colluded in a cover-up? Sure enough, research published this month in the *Lancet* has demonstrated a 'Cummings effect', a sharp and enduring decline in public confidence in the government's Covid strategy. The paper, from University College London, was based on more than 40,000 people's views of the government's approach to the pandemic, tracked over a six-week period.

I have neither the insider knowledge nor the expertise to pretend to understand the root causes of our world-beating mortality rate. It is all too soon, too overwhelming and complex. I am still prone to tears and insomnia. One day, a public inquiry presided over by a judge's cool eye will be called for, a forensic dissection far away from all this heat. However tempting it is to assign kneejerk blame now, those 65,000 excess deaths are clearly not an issue of poor political leadership alone. Number Ten's strategy was initially shaped and backed by senior experts guiding the government. On the podium, Johnson was invariably flanked by his chief medical and scientific advisers. The NHS, although widely regarded to have risen to the challenge, failed to foresee the dangers of the feverish rush to create hospital capacity. We are all, I believe – and it haunts me still – to some extent complicit in prioritising the expansion of hospital capacity above protecting the elderly, the vulnerable, the disabled and those with non-Covid diseases.

The Prime Minister's congratulatory NHS rhetoric is factu-
ally incorrect. We did *not* protect the NHS so much as turn it
off. We cancelled all non-urgent surgery and postponed many
cancer treatments. Yet, in the heat of the moment, were there
really any other practical options, given the hollowed-out state
of the health service after a decade's underfunding?

All this is for a future public inquiry to determine. For now,
though, I am reminded of a line from Rudyard Kipling. In a
speech to the Royal College of Surgeons in 1923, Kipling, who
once flirted with studying medicine before his squeamishness
got the better of him, stated: 'I am, by calling, a dealer in
words; and words are, of course, the most powerful drug used
by mankind.' No one knows this better than a palliative care
doctor. When drugs run dry, when cure is no longer an option,
I deal in words like my patients' lives depend on it. Words
build trust, allay fears, dispel myths, inspire hope. They clar-
ify, challenge, encourage and console. Words leap beyond the
constraints of masks and gloves and gowns. Titrated carefully,
dosed just right, words can take a dying patient all the way from
the depths of despair to a place of hope and even serenity. As
Kipling went on: 'Not only do words infect, egotise, narcotise,
and paralyse, but they enter into and colour the minutest cells of
the brain.' It follows that doctors have a duty to use our words
with exceptional care. We are nothing if our patients cannot
trust us. Above all, our word must be our bond.

Politicians are also expert wordsmiths, though the link
between the words they utter and the lives and deaths of the
people they serve is typically more convoluted. Cause, effect.
Easy to infer, much harder to prove. But these are atypical times.
In a pandemic, as in wartime, a nation's collective behaviour

clearly helps determine the ultimate death toll. Words drive behaviours drive dying. This basic fact of crisis governance was, of course, exploited brilliantly by Boris Johnson's idol, Winston Churchill, who famously mobilised the English language and sent it into battle.

Is it hopelessly naive, anachronistic even, to expect verbal sincerity and candour from today's politicians in calamitous times? 'I must level with you,' the Prime Minister told us early on, and I craved and needed that levelling. But in my darkest moments, I worry that all those televised Covid press conferences were used increasingly to distract us from what was really at stake. That the flood of pseudoscientific statistics was intended, primarily, to bamboozle – to leave the population dazed, bemused and therefore compliant. When you are invited daily to celebrate supersized statistics – 100,000 tests a day; no, make that 250,000 – it is easy to lose sight of what matters.

Sir David Spiegelhalter, Professor of the Public Understanding of Risk at Cambridge University, suggested in May that Downing Street was using 'number theatre' to manipulate the message rather than actually inform people. The chair of the UK Statistics Authority, Sir David Norgrove, was also forced to write to the health secretary, Matt Hancock, to urge him to improve the 'trustworthiness' of the way he presented data on coronavirus testing. Sometimes I would reel, punch drunk, from televised press conference to press conference, wondering whether those standing on the podium were seeking, above all, not to inform and educate but to gloss over recent history.

The true metric of success in a pandemic is simple: the overall number of deaths prevented. The point of our response to coronavirus was never to flatten curves, ramp up headlines, protect the NHS or invent mathematically nonsensical statistics: it was the prevention of unnecessary dying. It is a fact that our death toll is catastrophic, and that 400,000 of our most vulnerable citizens, those residing in care homes, were abandoned to Covid. We have not, in any sense, done well. And though mistakes in a pandemic are of course inevitable, deliberate misinformation is unforgivable.

In the end, does it really matter if the alleged 'success' of April came at such stupendous cost to those too elderly, frail or disabled to live in their own homes? You could argue – indeed, some commentators have essentially done so – that there was little point to the men and women I cared for as they died in their hospital beds from Covid. They were often people in their eighties and nineties who had not been economically productive for decades. They were lucky, weren't they, to have had an innings like that? Of course the young must come first. You might even have championed one old man's exploits – the charm, determination and ebullience of Captain Tom – while being secretly at peace with the expendability of certain parts of the herd.

To those of us up close to this dreadful disease – who have seen, as we have, the way it suffocates the life from you – such judgements are grotesque. The moment we rank life according to who most 'deserve' it, we have crossed into a realm I don't want to be a part of – and I struggle to believe many other Britons do either. The way out of a pandemic cannot, surely, entail the sacrifice of those deemed less worth saving?

Writing this now at the tail end of summer, I worry that people may not understand how very close the NHS came to being overwhelmed this Easter, how we avoided the hellishness of Lombardy and New York City only by superhuman efforts. I fear, too, that the public is unaware of how exhausted, stunned – shell-shocked, even – many NHS staff and care workers remain. How daunted we feel watching lockdown relax when proper testing, tracing and isolation infrastructure are still not in place. How incredulous we have been to see government figures breaking the rules they wrote, that so many others have lived and died by.

Shortly after the pandemic's Easter peak, nothing was more contagious than Covid battle rhetoric, not even the virus itself. Tobias Ellwood MP, chair of the House of Commons Defence Select Committee, took the language of war to new, literal heights with the suggestion that the Red Arrows and other military aircraft should raise the nation's morale by performing metropolitan flypasts during Thursday-evening 'claps for carers'. Being married to a former Royal Air Force fighter pilot, I know precisely how eloquent and moving a ceremonial flight can be – in particular, the military's 'missing man' formation. This aerial salute, usually in honour of a fallen comrade, involves one pilot within a small formation of aircraft abruptly pulling up and away from their fellows, vanishing symbolically into a blue vault of sky. It is impossible to watch without your heart unravelling.

But doctors, nurses and carers are not, typically, members of the armed forces. We signed up to save lives, not (when necessary) to kill. And the increasingly bombastic proposals for honouring our 'sacrifice' were beginning to feel more disconcerting than uplifting. It is easier, after all, to live with doctors and nurses being lost 'in action' once you have first depersonalised them as heroes. I never wanted Red Arrows, medals or minutes of silence. Like my colleagues, my needs were more prosaic. Really, I just wanted honesty from those who rule us, sufficient Covid testing and fit-for-purpose PPE. The irony, after all, could not have been lost on Boris Johnson that the one thing Hollywood scriptwriters reliably award their superheroes is, at least, a mask and cape?

I am sitting in the sunshine with Ken Wood, his wife Helen and their dog Bertie in the warmth and peace of their garden. The Woods have just returned from a family holiday, from which Ken sent me the following message: 'We're in Scotland, Rachel, where I'm enjoying mountain biking, walking and – especially – the fellowship and merriment around our family table. Both girls are here. This is a dream come true and an answer to many prayers.'

It is almost impossible to believe that this ruddy, exuberant man of sixty spent weeks close to death on a ventilator. Burnished and bronzed by the Scottish weather, the words 'rude health' were made for him. I shift in my chair as I awkwardly observe that I'm decidedly pasty in comparison. Prior to this holiday, while he recuperated at home from his time in ICU, Ken felt compelled to write to the team that saved him: 'ICU staff laboured with professionalism and care over my feeble, ventilated body. I experienced several days of recovery with the same team's gentleness, empathy, and encouragement ... Thanks to the care I received, I am restored to my family and community. I will never forget what has been done for me, and what staff continue to do for others ... I believe I have a second chance at life.'

Ken's recovery has not been problem-free. The act of driving across the Scottish border triggered one of several waves of sudden and engulfing terror. Abruptly, he was back in the delirious world of his intensive care psychosis, drenched with fear of being kidnapped and imprisoned. 'Four months on, the Covid tentacle still stretches out to touch me,' he tells me. But he is here. He is alive. He cannot contain his gratitude.

I smile as he tells me about his runs and cold showers, how he's not quite back to par but he's getting there. And I think to myself, *this*. This is what it was all about. This is what the doctors, nurses, porters, carers, midwives, radiologists, biomedical scientists, estate teams, dieticians, speech and language therapists, physiotherapists, psychologists, receptionists, telephonists and all the other healthcare professionals came to work to try to achieve. They stepped into the Covid streets and breathed in and out the Covid air for him – for Ken – for all those like him. And he knows it and will never forget it.

'I want to hold on to it for ever. I don't ever want to take anything for granted again. I want to savour the life I have before me. I want to *live*.'

References

Camus, A., *The Plague* (London: Penguin Classics, 2002).

Prologue

Bellow, S., *Humboldt's Gift* (London: Penguin, 1984).
Portions of the article '"This man knows he's dying as surely
    as I do": a doctor's dispatches from the NHS frontline'
    by Rachel Clarke originally appeared in the *Guardian*
    on 30 May 2020.

Pneumonia of Unknown Cause

Wells, H. G., *The War of the Worlds* (London: Penguin, 2018).
Green, A., 'Li Wenliang', *Lancet*, 18 February 2020.
Wilder-Smith, A., et al., 'Can we contain the COVID-19
    outbreak with the same measures as for SARS?', *Lancet*,
    1 May 2020.
Woo, P., et al., 'Infectious diseases emerging from Chinese
    wet-markets: zoonotic origins of severe respiratory
    viral infections', *Current Opinion in Infectious Diseases*, 30
    October 2006.

Triggle, N., et al., '11 charts on the problems facing the NHS', *BBC News*, 9 January 2020.

Huang, C., et al., 'Clinical features of patients infected with 2019 novel coronavirus in Wuhan, China', *Lancet*, 24 January 2020.

Boseley, S., 'China's Sars-like illness worries health experts', *Guardian*, 9 January 2020.

The Might of Tiny Things

Medawar, P. B. & Medawar, J. S., 'Viruses', in Medawar, P. B. & Medawar, J. S. (eds) *Aristotle to Zoos: A Philosophical Dictionary of Biology* (Cambridge: Harvard University Press, 1983).

Sehdev, P., 'The Origin of Quarantine', *Clinical Infectious Diseases*, 1 November 2002.

Brooks, S., et al., 'The psychological impact of quarantine and how to reduce it: rapid review of the evidence', *Lancet*, 26 February 2020.

'He warned of coronavirus. Here's what he told us before he died', *New York Times*, 7 February 2020.

Hancock, M., 'Statement on Wuhan Coronavirus to the House of Commons', *Parliament UK*, 11 February 2020.

Kupferschmidt, K., 'Discovered a disease? WHO has new rules for avoiding offensive names', *Science*, 11 May 2015.

Solnit, R., *Call Them by Their True Names: American Crises and Essays* (London: Granta, 2018).

Gregory, A., 'Coronavirus: Man racially abuses woman then

knocks her friend unconscious after she confronts him',
Independent, 24 February 2020.

Giordano, P., *How Contagion Works* (London: W&N, 2020).

Calvert, J., et al., 'Coronavirus: 38 days when Britain
sleepwalked into disaster', *Sunday Times*,
19 April 2020.

Conn, D., et al., 'Revealed: the inside story of the UK's
Covid-19 crisis', *Guardian*, 29 April 2020.

Worst-case Scenarios

Williams, W. C., *The Autobiography of William Carlos Williams*
(New York: New Directions, 1967).

Crawford, D., *Viruses: A Very Short Introduction* (Oxford:
Oxford University Press, 2018).

Johns Hopkins University, 'COVID-19 Dashboard by the
Center for Systems Science and Engineering (CSSE)',
Johns Hopkins University, accessed 8 March 2020.

Kington, T., 'Coronavirus: Doctors forced into life-or-death
decisions as patients swamp hospitals', *The Times*, 11
March 2020.

Williams, W. C., 'Spring and All', *The Collected Poems of
William Carlos Williams: Vol.1: 1909–1939* (New York:
New Directions, 1987).

Spinney, L., *Pale Rider: The Spanish Flu of 1918 and how it
Changed the World* (London: Jonathan Cape, 2017).

A Brilliant Plan

McCarthy, C., *The Road* (London: Picador, 2009).

Prague, J., https://twitter.com/julia_prague/
    status/1240611364797911041, 19 March 2020.

Silvey, N., https://twitter.com/silv24/
    status/1241447017945223169?lang=en,
    21 March 2020.

Archer, B., 'Boris Johnson braves coronavirus outbreak with
    pregnant fiancée to support England', *Daily Express*, 8
    March 2020.

Peston, R., 'British government wants UK to acquire
    coronavirus "herd immunity"', *ITV News*, 12
    March 2020.

Hunt, J., quoted in 'Coronavirus: UK measures defended
    after criticism', *BBC News*, 13 March 2020.

'Has the Government Failed the NHS?' *BBC Panorama*, 8
    April 2020.

A Long Deep Breath

Bostridge, M., *Florence Nightingale: The Woman and Her
    Legend* (London: Penguin, 2020).

Horton, R., 'Scientists have been sounding the alarm on
    coronavirus for months. Why did Britain fail to act?',
    Guardian, 18 March 2020.

Hunter, D., et al., 'Covid-19 and the Stiff Upper Lip – The
    Pandemic Response in the United Kingdom', *New
    England Journal of Medicine*, 16 April 2020.

Dunhill, L., 'Critical care unit overwhelmed by coronavirus
    patients', *Health Service Journal*, 20 March 2020.

Jones, D., https://twitter.com/WelshGasDoc/
    status/1241083898999771137, 20 March 2020.

References

Campbell, D., et al., 'London hospitals struggle to cope with coronavirus surge', *Guardian*, 20 March 2020.

Hopson, C., 'Confronting coronavirus in the NHS: The story so far', *NHS Providers*, 15 April 2020.

Cook, T., 'I'm an ICU doctor. The NHS isn't ready for the coronavirus crisis', *Guardian*, 3 March 2020.

COVID-19 Hospital Discharge Service Requirements, *HM Government*, 19 March 2020.

The Thin Red Line

Macdonald, H., *Vesper Flights* (London: Jonathan Cape, 2020).

'NHS confirms first death of a UK doctor due to coronavirus', *Pulse Today*, 30 March 2020.

Gibbons, K., 'Doctors forced to buy safety gear from DIY stores', *The Times*, 26 March 2020.

Hignett, K., '"I'm losing the will to live, god help us all": despair of NHS procurement chief', *Health Service Journal*, 30 March 2020.

Inside the Wave

Holleran, A., *Chronicle of a Plague, Revisited: AIDS and its Aftermath* (Philadelphia: Da Capo Press, 2008).

Litz, B. T., et al., 'Moral injury and moral repair in war veterans: A preliminary model and intervention strategy', *Clinical Psychology Review*, 29 December 2009.

St Joseph's Hospice, https://twitter.com/stjohospice/status/1244606136407470081, accessed 21 September 2020.

The Thing with Feathers

Cohen, L., 'Anthem', *The Future*, 1992.

Cochrane, A., *One Man's Medicine: An Autobiography of Professor Archie Cochrane* (London: British Medical Journal, 1989).

Portions of the article 'Palliative care: what I learnt from my patients about confronting human mortality' by Rachel Clarke originally appeared in the *Sunday Times* on 12 April 2020.

Dickinson, E., '"Hope" is the Thing With Feathers', *The Complete Poems of Emily Dickinson* (Cambridge: The Belknap Press, 1983).

Sacrifice

Palacio, R. J., *Wonder* (London: Corgi Childrens, 2014).

Smith, Z., *Intimations: Six Essays* (London: Penguin, 2020).

Abdul, G., 'Pandemic-baking Britain has an "obscene" need for flour', *New York Times*, 20 May 2020.

Emily Maitlis, *BBC Newsnight*, 9 April 2020.

Human Factors

Camus, A., *The Plague* (London: Penguin Classics, 2002).

Yerkes, R. M., et al., 'The relation of strength of stimulus to rapidity of habit-formation', *Journal of Comparative Neurology and Psychology*, 1908.

'Human Factors in Healthcare', *NHS England*, https://www.england.nhs.uk/wp-content/uploads/2013/11/

nqb-hum-fact-concord.pdf, accessed 21 September 2020.

Booth, R., 'GP calls for action after 125 of her care home patients die of Covid-19', *Guardian*, 22 April 2020.

Birrell, I., 'A callous betrayal of our most vulnerable: The care home coronavirus scandal goes into the bedrock of our society – the failure to protect our most frail ... in a system left to rot by our social care failure', *Daily Mail*, 14 April 2020.

'Coronavirus: "Earlier lockdown would have halved death toll"', *BBC News*, 10 June 2020.

Cave, N., *The Red Hand Files*, Issue 6, October 2018, https://www.theredhandfiles.com/communication-dream-feeling/, accessed 21 September 2020.

Epilogue

Heaney, S., *Beowulf* (London: Faber & Faber, 2000).

Portions of the article 'NHS doctor: Forget medals and flypasts – what we want is proper pay and PPE' by Rachel Clarke originally appeared in the *Observer* on 3 May 2020.

Lintern, S., 'Coronavirus: Deaths of hundreds of frontline NHS and care workers to be investigated', *Independent*, 11 August 2020.

Stafford, M., et al., 'Inequalities and deaths involving COVID-19: What the links between inequalities tell us', *Health Foundation*, 21 May 2020.

'Disparities in the risk and outcomes of COVID-19', *Public Health England*, Aug 2020.

de Prudhoe, K., 'My dad died alone because we played by
    the rules. Why is it different for Dominic Cummings?',
    Huffington Post, 26 May 2020.

Ellery, B., et al., 'Loyalty to Dominic Cummings will cost
    lives, says scientist', *The Times*, 25 May 2020.

Fancourt, D., et al., 'The Cummings effect: politics, trust,
    and behaviours during the COVID-19 pandemic',
    Lancet, 6 August 2020.

Canale, D. J., 'Rudyard Kipling's medical addresses', *Journal of
    Medical Biography*, 11 March 2019.

Spiegelhalter, D., *BBC Andrew Marr Show*, 10 May 2020.

Sir David Norgrove's response to Matt Hancock regarding
    the government's COVID-19 testing data, *UK Statistics
    Authority*, 2 June 2020.

Acknowledgements

Firstly, thank you to my magnificent agent, Clare Alexander, without whose faith, encouragement and unwavering eye this book would never have been written.

Huge thanks also to Richard Beswick, my wise and brilliant editor, and to Grace Vincent, Emily Moran, Nithya Rae, Ellen Rockwell, Daniel Balado and the rest of the wonderful team at Little, Brown whose enthusiasm and talents are second to none.

Thank you so much, Mark Haddon, Kathryn Mannix, Henry Marsh and Natasha Wiggins for sharing your time to read the draft and give so generously of your advice and wisdom.

Thank you to the many named and unnamed colleagues, patients and relatives who were kind enough to talk to me as part of my research for this book. I have tried my very hardest to do justice to your testimony.

I am lucky enough to work with an exceptionally kind and dedicated team of NHS and hospice colleagues who inspire me daily. Special thanks to Charlie Bond, Beth MacGregor, Ros Henderson, Julia Bartley, Victoria Hedges, Mandi Kitching, Helen Fletcher, Nic Rossiter, Angharad Orchard, Tracey Allen, Mel Moreton, Fiona Smith, Sarah Challis, Fiona Moore, Geraldine O'Meara, Holly Armstrong, Susan Chambers,

James Grote, Sarah Slatter, Justyna Rzońca, Chrissie Earle, Tina Griffin, Lisa Rayner, Sue Oxley, Caroline Whitford, Debbie Pay, Karen Nurse, Hannah Mozelewski and Nicki Tout. Thanks also to the amazing friends and colleagues I wish I worked with still, especially Christina Lovell, Rochelle Lay, Damian Choma, Abbie Hessey, Jane Henderson, Natasha Wiggins, Farzana Virani, Sarah Hanrott, Mary Miller, Tim Harrison, Andy King, Tim Littlewood and John Reynolds.

To my patients, from whom I learn so much – and for whom it is my privilege to care – my deepest thanks.

And finally, to dearest Dave, Finn and Abbey, thank you for surviving lockdown without me, and for unfailingly filling me hope and happiness.